Dr Alexander Logan

Get Me Into Medical School! Series

Should I Become A Doctor?

© Meddicle Publishing 2014
www.getmeintomedicalschool.com

Cover design by A Logan
Book design by A Logan
Character design by G Young

ISBN: 978-0-9931138-0-2

Get Me Into Medical School! Series

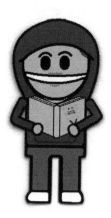

www.getmeintomedicalschool.com

Introduction

" Should I become a doctor?"

Deciding what to study at university is a tough decision to make. The question of 'what do you want to be?' is even more difficult when posed by teachers, parents, friends or relatives.

People want to become doctors for a variety of reasons including to gain respect, exposure to role models, family pressures, wanting to help others, financial rewards and love of practical skills.

You may have seen doctors portrayed by television shows and movies as smart and attractive, driving fast cars and attending decadent parties, however, in reality night shifts and busy on call periods are far from a luxury lifestyle.

Medicine is a fantastic career and doctors are some of the most trusted members of society, able to offer hope and comfort to patients in times of injury and ill health.

With this privilege of being invited into patients' lives comes a weight of responsibility not seen in many other careers. Medicine is extremely rewarding when patients do well following treatment but can be emotionally draining when they do not.

This book aims to give you all the information you need (plus some information you might not have considered) to help you decide whether you wish to study medicine in the United Kingdom and become a doctor.

The book draws on the experiences over over fifty medical professionals and offers virtual work experience together with insider facts that you might have had difficulty finding such as 'how much are doctors paid?', 'do I have to work every Christmas?' and 'what happens after I graduate from medical school?'.

Whatever decision you make after reading this book we hope that you select a career that you enjoy and look forward to going into work everyday.

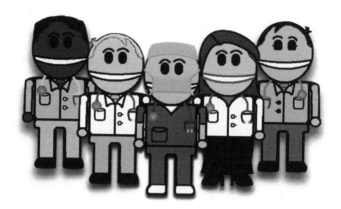

Chapter 1: Is Medicine The Course For Me?

Before applying it is important that you are 100% sure that medicine is the course for you. You will be in the same region for at least five years of undergraduate training before graduating and undertaking the foundation programme and then specialty training.

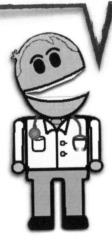

IS MEDICINE FOR ME?

Before applying to medical school the first step is to ensure that you definitely want to study medicine at university. Chances are that if you have picked up this book you are fairly sure already, however, owing to the length and cost of studying medicine it is important that you have sufficient information about the pros and cons of studying medicine before submitting your UCAS application.

Know What You Want

The first step is to think about what you would like from a career. This can be a daunting question and many people change careers a number of times in their lifetime as their immediate and longterm goals change. It is advisable to think about what you enjoy doing at the moment. Are you someone who enjoys learning new things? Do you enjoy science-based subjects? Do you enjoy practical tasks? Do you enjoy working with others? Do you enjoy working under pressure? Do you want responsibility?

Career choices are greatly influenced by role models and it is important that you look at people around you to see if they enjoy their jobs, are respected and are financially comfortable. Your personality type might also draw you towards a certain career. Our advice is to gain work experience in medicine but also in alternative careers that may interest you such as Law, Finance, Dentistry or others, this will help to ensure you are making the correct decision and limit the 'grass-is-greener' feeling when things may get tough in your chosen career.

Understanding yourself and your own goals is key to deciding whether a career in medicine will bring you a happy and fulfilling life or whether you are more suited to an alternative career.

Being Selfish and External Influences

Be completely honest with yourself and think hard about both the selfish and selfless reasons for wanting to study medicine. Put aside any pressures from school, peers or parents and think about your true motivations, you may even like to write these down. There is nothing 'bad' about wanting to be called a Dr or about having a stable, respected, well-paid job however if these are the only reasons for choosing medicine you need to ensure that you will enjoy going into work everyday, enjoy lifelong learning and do not mind earning less in the early years than your peers in city banking or dentistry. Equally if you fall into the old personal statement adage of 'wanting to help people' without any other motivations it is important that you realise there are many careers that help people such as charity workers, nurses or physios with shorter degree courses.

ATTRIBUTES OF A DOCTOR

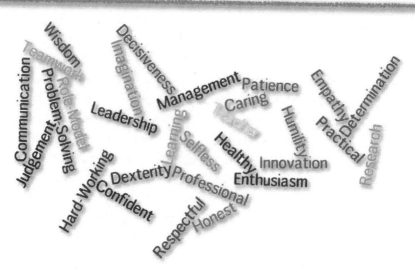

The General Medical Council (GMC) outlines the attributes required of a doctor. It is important that you possess at least some of these qualities already with the remainder learned and developed during medical school.

Six attributes that you should already possess include:

Intelligence Gaining three As in science-based subjects can be challenging and a strong academic ability is a necessity when learning about diseases, drug interactions and anatomy during medical school and in clinical practice.

Caring It is important that you want to help others as patient-centred care is at the core of modern medicine. A caring healthcare system is particularly topical following the recommendations of The Francis Report and Mid-Staffs Enquiry in 2013.

Determination Medicine is a long degree course and postgraduate training requires moving hospitals and paying for mandatory courses. It is important that you are focussed and determined to reach the end.

Communication Skills One of the best aspects of medicine is the opportunity to interact with a variety of both patients and colleagues. Eliciting medical histories from patients and co-ordinating treatment plans with the multidisciplinary team require being able to communicate effectively.

Dexterity Whether it is listening to heart sounds or performing a total hip replacement medicine involves performing practical procedures. Having a natural affinity for manual tasks will be of great help when putting in a difficult cannula or taking blood from an unwell patient.

Common Sense While facts and evidence from your medical training will often point you towards the most appropriate course of action or diagnosis much of medicine comes from sound judgement and making sensible choices when presented with management options or ethical dilemmas.

Insider Opinions From Students and Doctors

Insider's Edge 1

" Being honest with myself I chose medicine as I believed I would be a high-earner. While I was determined to get into the competitive degree course and did so, I found the necessity to move around hospitals, sometimes living in meagre accommodation, and having to sit postgraduate exams unrewarding.

I took the decision to leave medicine following completion of my core surgical training years, aged 28, to pursue a career in city banking and business. I was happy to see that my medical training and skills were well-received in the city and I was able to use my creativity to set up a business which rewards me with more freedom to enjoy life.

I firmly believe that I was fixated on the competitive entry and perceived status of becoming a doctor without having understood what life was really like due to inadequate work experience. "

Insider's Edge 2

" I had always wanted to be a TV presenter but after seeing a friend's older brother working as a doctor I decided to undertake work experience at my local hospital. I found the experience amazing and, although still not 100% certain, I applied to medical school and have never looked back since. Few careers marry practical skills with investigative skills and reward you by helping people get better. As a Trauma and Orthopaedic surgeon I can now help people with severe immobility due to osteoarthritis to walk pain free with hip or knee replacements and can also instantly identify injuries on X-rays, operate to fix them on the same day and then send the patient home within a 48 hour period. There is also plenty of

private practice to ensure my wife and children are well looked-after! "

Insider's Edge 3

" My family are all doctors and I knew that medical training was long but rewarding and knew that my parents enjoyed their jobs. Despite this after qualifying I realised that I hated night shifts and working weekends. It was difficult socialising during the week as either I was working or my friends were working making meeting up challenging.
I decided to do GP training for this reason and after three years of training am now self-employed and able to take time off when I want and don't have to work night shifts or weekends unless I want to earn some

more money as a locum doctor filling in a rota slot. "

THE POSITIVES AND NEGATIVES OF MEDICINE

The Negatives	The Positives
• People die/blood and guts	• Saving/changing lives
• High-pressure	• High-pressure
• Competitive at all levels	• Well-respected
• Long course	• Job security and well-paid
• Long postgraduate training	• Multiple career paths
• Financial commitment	• Variety of patients and diseases
• Private work only as consultant	• Intellectually challenging
• Cost-cutting and bad press	• Develops leadership skills
• Lots of exams	• Lifelong learning and improvement
• Shift work/working nights	• Able to teach junior colleagues
• Moving around hospitals	• Practical and technical skills

Insider's Edge 4

" Medicine can be tough but it can also be very rewarding.

The worst parts about medicine are having to move around hospitals for undergraduate and postgraduate training and sometimes living in areas that you might not choose to live yourself for the sake of work. Night shifts and weekends can limit your social time when you qualify and you can become envious of friends in the private sector who seem to have more free time and earn more money in the fist few years. In reality you will be working fewer hours per week than private sector workers and will likely have time off after nights. The variety of both patients and procedures makes the job much more interesting than office work though the responsibility is not for everyone. "

MEDICAL TRAINING OVERVIEW

Medical School (4-6 years) Most UK medical courses last five years (four for accelerated graduate programmes and six if you undertake an intercalated degree). Courses may be traditional (preclinical lecture-based teaching then clinical years) or integrated (lectures and patient contact from day one). Each teaching style has pros and cons and this is explored in more in Chapter 4 Choosing a Medical School.

Foundation Years (2 years) Following graduation and gaining the title of 'Dr' graduates undertake the two-year foundation programme. This consists of six four-month placements covering medicine and surgical specialties and designed to give doctors a grounding for identifying and treating medical and surgical patients. Following the F1 year doctors become fully registered with the GMC.

Core Training/Specialty Training (3-10 years) Eighteen months into Foundation training doctors can apply for core or specialty training. The selection process and training periods differ between specialties with GP training lasting three years and medical and surgical specialties requiring two years of core training followed by selection into higher specialist training at ST3 level. Some specialties such as radiology offer so-called run-through posts with no competition for posts at ST3 level effectively 'running through' from the end of F2 to consultant posts.

Consultant Posts Following specialist training and completion of any exit examinations doctors receive their certificate for completion of training (CCT) and may apply for a consultant post in their chosen specialty. Most consultants are around thirty-two to thirty-five at the time of their appointment and may then undertake private practice.

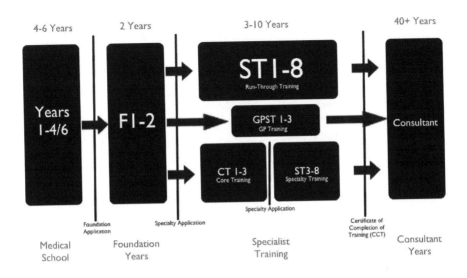

A more comprehensive look at life as a medical student, foundation doctor and in specialty training can be found in Chapter 2. It is highly recommended you read this chapter as it will enhance and focus your work experience together with providing ammunition for interview questions.

It is also important to remember that medicine is constantly changing, in five years 50% of medical knowledge will have altered in some form, and this applies to training too. Interviews, length of training and roles of doctors are under constant scrutiny from both the department of health and the Royal Colleges (who are responsible for postgraduate training). One example is the three year GP training programme which may be extended to five years in the near future.

How Much Will I Get Paid As A Doctor?

While some refrain from talking about doctor's salaries we feel that it is vital future medics have as much information about medicine as possible before making an informed career choice.

There have been a number of changes to doctors salaries over the past decade brought on by economic pressure, reforms to medical training and a reduction in working hours. While the overall trend has been a downward one, this has also come with a reduction in working hours from upwards of 80 hours per week to 48 hours per week improving both patient safety and work-life balance.

Calculating a doctor's salary can be difficult as together with the basic salaries outlined below pay is affected by an hours-worked multiplier known as 'banding'. If the doctor is contracted to work more than 40 hours and/or to work outside 7am-7pm Monday to Friday, they will receive an additional supplement which will normally be between 20% and 50% of basic salary. This supplement is based on the extra hours worked above a 40 hour standard working week and the intensity of the work.

For example an F2 doctor earning a base salary of £27K a year while on a surgical job banded at 50% would effectively be earning closer to £40K a year for his/her time in that job.

Foundation Year 1 £22,412 basic salary (£1800/month after tax)

Foundation Year 2 £27,798 basic salary (£2200/month after tax)

Specialty Training £29,705 basic salary increasing per year of training (£2500-£2800/month after tax)

General Practitioners between £53,781 to £81,158 basic salary (£2800-£4000/month after tax)

In addition GPs can gain supplements by meeting set targets, housing a private pharmacy on their premises, undertaking private practice and working as 'locums'.

Hospital Consultant between £74,504 and £100,446 basic NHS salary per year. Along with their yearly NHS salary consultants may add supplementary wages:

Consultants are eligible for bonuses from clinical excellence awards if they meet targets.

Consultants may undertake private work outside of the NHS.

Consultants may take on roles within a hospital or trust such as clinical director which come with more work but an additional salary in the region of £80-100K per year.

WHAT HOURS WILL I WORK?

Due to the reduction in working hours there is a limit of 48 hours of work per week. This effectively means that most junior doctors work a 9-5 or 8-5 shift pattern with intermittent days or weekends of 'on call' when they work a longer 12 hour shift.

Hours and shift patterns are dependent on the specialty. For most specialties, doctors work 3 weekends, 15 on call days and 3 weeks of night shifts (8pm to 8am) per four months. Night shifts often come with a week off work afterwards and doctors are entitled to 28 days of annual leave per year and 28 days of study leave to attend courses or exams per year.

As medicine is shift-based using a rota you will often need to give 6-8 weeks notice to take annual leave so that cover for your absence can be arranged.

Chapter 2: Life In Medicine

Medicine is a fantastic and varied career. The scope of medicine is so large that it can be difficult to appreciate all the different subspecialties and roles. This chapter is a great place to start before entering a hospital for work experience.

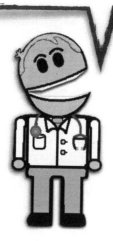

BEING A MEDICAL STUDENT

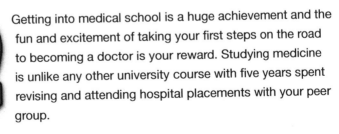

Getting into medical school is a huge achievement and the fun and excitement of taking your first steps on the road to becoming a doctor is your reward. Studying medicine is unlike any other university course with five years spent revising and attending hospital placements with your peer group.

Medical school is vastly different from your experiences at school or on previous degree courses. The combination of practical, anatomical and problem-solving skills that you will be taught makes for a constantly evolving and challenging learning environment.

This chapter gives you a feel for what life is like as a medical student and offers some tips from current medical students to help you stay ahead.

Before You Start

Once you have accepted an offer at your chosen medical school you will be sent lots of information to prepare you for starting the course. Below are some things you may need to organise.

Immunisations It is a mandatory requirement that your immunisations are up to date before beginning clinical work. You will also need to have a Hep B immunisation. The medical school will send you a list of the required immunisations which can be completed at your GP surgery or with the university occupational health before starting the course.

Accommodation One of the first things you will want to organise is where you will live. Most universities will have an accommodation website with halls of residence, colleges or links to city residences. As with the UCAS form it is best to get your accommodation preferences sorted early to avoid disappointment.

Books Universities will often send you comprehensive reading lists with large textbooks. It is not advisable spending lots of money buying books before you start. Fellow students will often recommend the best textbooks and medical school libraries are well-stocked. Below are a selection of the most popular medical reference texts:

Kumar, P. and Clark, M. *Kumar and Clark Clinical Medicine*, Saunders, London.

Longman, M et al. *The Oxford Handbook of Clinical Medicine*, OUP, Oxford.

Drake, R. Vogl, W. and Mitchell, A. *Gray's Anatomy for Students*, Churchill Livingstone, London.

Moore, K. and Dalley, A. *Clinically Orientated Anatomy*, Lippincott Williams and Wilkins, Baltimore.

Apps There are lots of medical apps available and many medical textbooks are also offered in Kindle or iBook format. Anatomy flashcards and quick reference apps can be extremely useful when on hospital placement. The App Store is filled with thousands of medical applications and you will often be recommended useful apps by fellow students and lecturers. Below are a selection of the best:

Instant Anatomy Flash Cards Andrew Whitaker These hand-drawn anatomy annotations are a great quick-reference guide and are invaluable when cramming for anatomy spot tests.

Gray's Anatomy Flash Cards Drake, R et al. A compact version of the well-known textbook makes it more accessible and fun.

Oxford Handbook of Clinical Medicine OUP The app version of the OHCM is a natural replacement for students carrying the (almost) pocket-size book with them on the wards.

Medical Gear The most important things to take with you for clinical placements are smart clothes and a stethoscope. Most medical schools will offer a Littmann stethoscope to new students at a discounted price (RRP £60).

Your First Week (Freshers' Week)

Your first week of university will be amazing. You will meet many new friends from both your medical course and from your halls of residence or college. The first week will begin with an introduction to university life with welcome events and nights-out organised for new students. You will also be required to register at the medical school and the university precinct if you have not done so already.

The medical school will send you a timetable and will usually feature a week of introductory lectures and events to help you get to know the medical school and your fellow students.

Walking into your accommodation, meeting room mates and sitting down in lectures for the first time can be scary but it is also exciting and you will meet lots of new people. Our advice is to talk to everyone. Everyone is new to the university and it is a great opportunity to meet as many people as possible.

Getting Organised

After a week of new experiences and enjoying yourself it can be easy to forget that you are at medical school to learn medicine. It is important that you get on top of your studies from the first term. Studying at university is much more self-directed and you will be expected to work in your own time and read around lecture topics. It is also important that you keep yourself organised with a calendar containing assignment deadlines and examination dates. Below are some top tips on how to keep on top of your work while also enjoying yourself:

File Your Notes At the start of the year buy yourself some A4 binders (one for each subject area). Store your lecture notes in these as you go along.

Most students spend hours sifting through disorganised notes just before exam periods before finally relenting to organisation.

Use a Calendar Apple iCal or other electronic calendars are a great way to keep on top of deadlines, holidays and exam dates.

Use the Facilities Your medical school will have a designated medical library, anatomy department and IT facilities for you to use. Make sure you know how to access these and get in the habit of using the quiet environment of the library to revise around exams.

Ask for Help Both your peers and lecturers will be happy to help explain any topics that you are struggling with. Don't be afraid to ask.

The Early Years (1-2)

As a First Year (Fresher) medical student you will likely spend most of your time in lectures or small groups discussing scenarios and cases. Your day will usually run from 9am to 5pm and be based at the medical school campus. You may also have tutorials in physiology, biochemistry and anatomy laboratories and venture out into GP practices and hospitals for the occasional clinical attachment.

	AM		PM
Monday	Physiology Lectures	Lunch	Biochemistry Lectures
Tuesday	Small Group Tutorials	Lunch	Communication Skills
Wednesday	Anatomy Labs	Lunch	Sports
Thursday	GP Attachment	Lunch	Anatomy Lectures
Friday	Core Medicine Lectures	Lunch	Pathology Lectures

Lectures usually last 45 minutes and a morning session is composed of between 2 and 4 lectures. Lectures break at 1-2pm for lunch. The days with 3 lectures in the afternoon can drag on while the more interesting days have anatomy or a practical sessions. After lectures most students head back to their accommodation for food before heading back out into the city for some socialising.

The Later Years (3-5)

As you progress though medical school you will be exposed to more and more clinical placements. Learning and working in a hospital environment is very different from any other type of study. Patients will happily allow you to examine them and partake in their care for your learning. It is important that you dress and act as a doctor would when on the wards, in clinic or in theatre.

	AM		PM
Monday	Clinic	Lunch	Free Study
Tuesday	Tutorial	Lunch	Ward Work
Wednesday	Ward Round	Lunch	Sports
Thursday	Clinic	Lunch	Tutorial
Friday	Tutorial	Lunch	Free Study

Most hospital placement focus on a specific specialty such as old age medicine, orthopaedic surgery or ophthalmology. You will visit a number of different specialties and departments to build up your skill-set of identifying and managing common diseases. Surgical specialties begin at 8am while medical specialties start with a ward round at 9am. Unless you are shadowing an 'on call' shift doctor you will be expected to work from 8/9am to 5pm. Your teaching will be a mix of ward and clinic based patient exposure and focused teaching sessions from clinicians.

Intercalation

Intercalate means to 'add between' and refers to medical students taking a year out of the medical course to study a different subject for a year and attain an extra undergraduate degree.

Different universities offer different subjects to intercalate in and the degree awarded is typically a BSc (Bachelor of Science) or BA (Bachelor of Arts).

Intercalation is optional and there are pros and cons to studying for an extra year. The most important deciding factor should be that you find the subject interesting.

Who can Intercalate? Intercalation is optional at most medical schools (See the Med Schools Guide Chapter for those with compulsory intercalated years) and, provided you have achieved a good academic standing in your first two years, anyone may intercalate.

When? Most students intercalate following years two or three of medical school.

Where? Most students that decide to intercalate choose to do so at their own university. If you wish to study for a year at a different university you may do so providing you get approval from the medical school.

Why? The best reason to choose to intercalate is that you are genuinely interested in the subject. Gaining an extra degree scores you a few points on the Foundation application but is not as useful for specialty selection where most applicants have postgraduate degrees such as a Masters' (MSc).

Why Not? The most obvious reasons are the cost of an extra year of study together with dropping back a year group. Once you graduate there is no difference between those with and those without an extra degree (apart from maybe their debt).

What Subjects? Each university has a list of intercalated degrees available. If there is a particular subject that is offered by another university you may apply to change to that university for your intercalated year before returning to your medical course.

Exams

Exams at medical school will be very different from those you have experienced at school or on previous degree courses. Revision is much more self-directed and it is important that you keep your notes organised and hit the library for three-four weeks before major exams.

MCQs Multiple choice question papers usually take the form of single best answer (SBA) and extended matching questions (EMQs) and are used to test core knowledge. SBAs provide you with a statement or question and ask you to select the most appropriate answer from a list of five potential answers. EMQs provide you with a list of ten potential answers and ask you to match a short sentence or paragraph to the most appropriate one. MCQ papers usually last two and a half hours and test core knowledge. The best way to pass them is to practise past papers.

Anatomy Spot This will take place in the anatomy department and will feature a selection of cadaveric or model pro-sections with structures labelled with numbers or letters. You will rotate around, spending one to two minutes with each prosection and will be asked to label structures on your question paper and answer clinical questions related to their function.

OSCE The objective structured clinical examination is similar to the MMI interview format. Medical school OSCEs test examination technique, history taking, practical skills and communication skills. You will rotate around ten to fifteen stations and will have five minutes to complete the desired task in each. OSCEs usually involve actors for communication stations and real patients for examination stations.

Long Case Your ability to take a history and examine a patient will be scrutinised by two examiners on a ward. During the early years this might focus on one particular system while for finals it resembles a driving test asking you to take a full history and examine all the body systems before suggesting a potential diagnosis.

Extracurricular

Although medicine is a tough subject and there will be lots of work there is plenty of time for you to pursue interests outside of medicine. Universities have a multitude of clubs and societies for you to join and medics often have their own sports and social teams. Joining teams and clubs is a great way to make friends, relax and put any worries in perspective. Having non-medical friends can be invaluable around revision time and during clinical attachments when medics tend to become quite intense.

Support

Medical schools usually adopt a parenting or buddy system with older medics looking after First year students. Medical 'parents' can be a great sources of advice and help if you are unsure about anything when you start.

The medical school and university will also offer a range of support services if you are struggling with any aspect of university life or the medical course.

Further Information

To find out exactly what your course, medical school and university offers make sure you take a good look at their medical school website. The admissions page will often give a full breakdown of the university course and offer insights from current students.

BEING A FOUNDATION DOCTOR

In the final year of medical school you will be asked to apply to the Foundation Programme. The two year Foundation Programme offers a general grounding in the basics of working as a hospital doctor before undertaking specialisation.

The Foundation Programme was introduced as part of the Modernising Medical Careers programme in 2006-7. Previously doctors in their first year after graduating undertook a Preregistration House Officer (PRHO) year, covering general medicine and general surgery, and then became a Senior House Officer (SHO) for two to three years in a set specialty before becoming a Registrar and then a Consultant.

Year 1	Year 2	Year 3	Year 4	Year 5-9	Year 10
F1	F2	ST/CT1	ST/CT2	ST3-8	Consultant
PRHO		SHO		Registrar	Consultant

Confusingly some medics still refer to F2 and ST/CT1-2 doctors as SHOs and this term is often used interchangeably for doctors more senior than F1 but not yet a Registrar (ST3).

There are 25 Foundation Schools located in 14 medical 'Deaneries'. A Deanery is a local area responsible for medical training. Recruitment to the Foundation Programme is a national process and you may apply to any of the 25 Foundation Schools within the United Kingdom. While individual job rotations and hospitals may differ the overall job is the same.

Foundation Year 1

The first of the two foundation years gives doctors an introduction to hospital medicine. F1 doctors rotate through three four-month placements and are the first point of contact for nursing staff. F1s are responsible for ensuring ward jobs are completed and ill patients are identified and flagged up to senior colleagues.

At the end of the F1 year doctors become fully registered with the General Medical Council (GMC) and gain full prescription rights.

Foundation Year 2

F2s take on more responsibility and often fit into on-call rotas with ST/CT1-2 doctors (the old SHO grade rota). Applications and interviews for the first step of specialty training open around Christmas time of the F2 year and so most doctors spend a lot of their free time polishing their CVs and undertaking audits, presentations or publications to maximise their chances of selection.

Further information on the foundation programme can be found here: www.foundationprogramme.nhs.uk

The Work Load

Foundation Doctors typically begin their day with a consultant or registrar-led ward-round. Depending on the specialty this might be quick (surgery) or very long (old age medicine). The F1/2 will keep a record of any jobs the consultant asks to be done on the ward round and will then spend the rest of the day completing them and troubleshooting any problems from the ward patients.

Depending on the job there will be an opportunity to attend clinic, perform diagnostic procedures (such as chest aspirations, lumbar punctures etc) or assist in theatre. The main responsibility of the F1/2 is to the ward patients and due to increasing hospital bureaucracy much of their time is spent completing electronic discharge summaries, writing drug charts or labelling pro-formas. F1/2s work as part of a team and time management and delegation tasks plays a large role in ensuring that the boring and fun jobs are shared equally.

F1/2s typically work three weekends and two-three weeks of nights with fourteen long-day on calls within each four month placement. Some placements such as A&E or Acute Medicine are more shift based. They may take nine days of annual leave for each four month placement and may take an additional fifteen days of study leave over the year.

Assessments

As with all of medicine Foundation doctors are continuously assessed to maintain patient safety. All F1/2s must maintain an online tool called the 'ePortfolio' up to date with reflective practice and feedback from colleagues. The ePortfolio is assessed at the end of the year and provided it has been maintained to an acceptable standard the doctor may progress to the following year. Throughout the year Foundation Doctors have a clinical and educational supervisor, usually a consultant in the specialty they are currently working in. The supervisor offers help and support with any problems and gives feedback through the ePortfolio on the Doctor's performance.

The Best and Worst of The Foundation Years

The Best	The Worst
• Experience many specialties	• Loads of paperwork
• Lots of new things to learn	• Jobs can be very busy
• More responsibility	• Even with shadowing your first day will be scary
• Get to help patients	• Pay not as high as dentistry or private-sector jobs
• You will be paid	
• Job security	• Shift-work can make socialising tricky

MEDICAL SUB-SPECIALTIES

Medicine is incredibly varied with a subspecialty of doctor for every system of the body. During medical school you will rotate through almost all of these specialties and gain an appreciation for what it is like being a doctor specialising in each area.

Selecting a career path can be a difficult decision. As you have already heard doctors must choose a specialist training post during their F2 year, 18 months after graduating from medical school. This does not leave much time for experiencing what it is like to work as a doctor in your desired specialty and Foundation doctors utilise 'taster days' (a work experience day for foundation doctors) and career events to gain insight into life in different medical careers.

For the more competitive areas such as surgery and anaesthetics it is important that doctors make their choice early and begin to build their CVs with audits, research, presentations and show commitment to that specialty. For less competitive careers there is often time to work abroad or as a locum and gain more experience of other specialties.

How to Choose

So how do you choose? Below we discuss some things you may wish to consider when thinking about a final career and we also explore some of the career options available to doctors.

Motivating Factors

It is likely that you will enjoy many different specialties during medical school and the Foundation years and your long term career plans may change on multiple occasions.

Personality Type Research has shown that even before medical school some students show a preponderance for certain careers based on their personalities. Career-driven males often favour surgery while others may favour the more relaxed idea of general practice. Make sure that you think beyond your gut and consider all factors

Role Models When on work experience, taster days or simply in the hospital make sure you pinpoint who enjoys their job and who you can relate to. Is there a doctor who you look up to or you could see yourself becoming?

Work-Life Balance Your priorities will change as you get older and while you may be very career driven at the moment you may wish to spend more time with your family in the future. Make sure you know how frequently doctors in each specialty are on call, work weekends, work nights and how busy their day-to-day job is.

Competition Application to specialty training is competitive and for surgeons and anaesthetists it can be very stressful with no guarantees of a job. If you are prepared to work hard and accept that you may need to reapply the following year this shouldn't be a problem, however, if you seek a more relaxed lifestyle GP or psychiatry may be a better choice.

Training The length and cost of training in each specialty differs greatly. GP training is short and inexpensive while surgery takes eight years and asks trainees to spend money on courses and exams. Conversely training is fun and a longer training period will make you more confident when you become a consultant.

Private Practice Most consultants gain extra income from private work on top of their NHS salaries. Some specialties, such as surgery, have a steady stream of private work and surgeons can make a healthy profit. The extra work, responsibility and insurance payments required by private work may put off the less financially motivated.

Research If you enjoy research at medical school you may wish to become an academic medic in a subspecialty. Some subspecialties have more of an emphasis on research than others and if you don't enjoy research projects you may wish yo avoid these.

The Job Make sure you know what doctors in your desired specialty do on a daily basis. Some specialties involve lots of practical procedures, some focus on the care of dying patients and some involve being based in a lab or office. Think about what you want to do for the next forty years.

Further Information on applying to medical specialties can be found here:

https://www.mmc.nhs.uk

Types of Career

In the next few sections we will look in detail at the career paths of some of the more popular specialties: physician, surgeon, GP and anaesthetist. It is important to remember that there are loads of opportunities to do extra work or think outside the box with your medical degree. Below are a few other ways to use your medical degree:

Academic Medicine Research and teaching is a large part of the medical community. As a doctor there are opportunities to undertake MSc, PhD or MD projects at medical research departments in the UK and abroad. Research can be laboratory based or clinical and consultants with a keen interest in research can become Professors and head university research departments. If you are more interested in teaching you may wish to become a lecturer at your university and teach the next generation of medical students.

Expedition Medicine Practising medicine is not just limited to hospitals. Many expeditions to tropical and dangerous locations will require medical support. As a qualified doctor you may undertake Wilderness and Expedition Medicine training in remote environments such as Jungle, Polar, Desert, Altitude or Underwater. Expedition medics are usually part of a team providing medical support to commercial or charity organisations travelling in hostile environments.

Medical Entrepreneur Some medics have great ideas that could improve patient safety or translate into a commercially viable business. You could invent a surgical tool, develop a website or set up a charity.

Working Abroad You can take your medical degree virtually anywhere in the world. Many junior doctors head to Australia following their Foundation Year 2 year before applying to specialist training. Both the US and Canada require all foreign doctors to successfully pass medical licensing examinations before applying for work and these are similar to the exams you will sit during medical school.

Locum Work Some doctors prefer the freedom that 'locuming' offers. Being a locum doctor essentially means that you are not in a training post but instead fill in gaps in rotas or in GP practices on an ad-hoc basis. Covering gaps in different specialties can be well paid but lacks job security and the training opportunities granted by traditional hospital posts. In reality many doctors do this while they are still deciding upon their chosen career path or on top of their day job to gain some extra cash.

BEING A PHYSICIAN

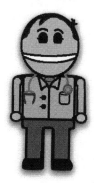

Physicians or 'medics' are the core medical doctors of the hospital. Physicians learn to recognise disease signs and symptoms and use their clinical acumen to diagnose and treat patients with medical illnesses.

The Royal College of Physicians defines their role as 'specialists in the diagnosis and treatment of medical conditions'. Physicians are interested in the general medical specialties such as Cardiology, Respiratory, Gastroenterology, Neurology, Endocrinology, Rheumatology, Dermatology and Old Age Medicine.

What Physicians Do

Medical doctors use their clinical history and examination skills to identify and manage medical conditions. Medical patients make up the majority of hospital inpatients and medical doctors can be very busy assessing new patients and looking after patients on medical wards.

The scope of medicine is vast with 26 subspecialties identified by the Royal College of Physicians (see below). This leads to much variety in their work with no two patients the same. Medics enjoy the challenge of diagnosing and treating diseases and medical doctors actively involve themselves in the multidisciplinary rehabilitation of patients before discharging them home.

Most hospitals have a Medical Admissions Unit run by acute medicine Consultants who work with an on call Registrar and team of Core Medical Trainees and Foundation Doctors to assess every new patient admitted to hospital through A&E, or directly from their GP, with a suspected medical condition. It is the role of the acute medical team to identify and treat any life-threatening conditions, start treatment and then send the patient to an appropriate medical subspecialty ward.

The medical 'take' (patients admitted to hospital) is usually much busier than surgery or other hospital specialties and on call medical doctors must continuously see and assess patients during their eight-hour shift.

Once a patient has been stabilised by the acute medical team they will then be seen on a specialty ward by the appropriate medical team.

Example: A 92 year old man is admitted to hospital from a nursing home with increasing confusion, a temperature and a productive cough. The acute medical team take some bloods and perform a chest X-ray which confirms an upper lobe pneumonia and start the patient on IV antibiotics and some fluids. As he remains stable and he is from a nursing home he is transferred to a care of the elderly ward to be looked after by the specialist team.

In this way a patient with a heart condition can be transferred to a cardiology ward or a patient with a pneumothorax to a respiratory ward to ensure that they receive expert care.

On specialist medical wards the medical team is composed of a Consultant, a medical registrar a core medical trainee and one or two foundation doctors. The day usually begins with a long ward round of all the patients on the ward with the F1 pushing a notes trolley around the bays. The consultant identifies any tests that need doing or changes to a patient's treatment and teaches the more junior team members.

It is not all acute medicine, however. Physicians also run clinics to follow up patients with chronic medical conditions in the community. Some medical specialties such as dermatology or rheumatology are almost all clinic-based with no inpatients and virtually all patients managed as outpatients. This can be a nice lifestyle for people who enjoy specialising in an area and would prefer not to become GPs.

Subspecialties

The Royal College of Physicians has identified 30 subspecialties within medicine. They are:

Acute Medicine	Infectious Diseases
Allergy	Medical Oncology
Audiological Medicine	Medical Ophthalmology
Cardiology	Metabolic Medicine
Clinical Genetics	Neurology
Clinical Neurophysiology	Nuclear Medicine
Clinical Pharmacology and Therapeutics	Paediatric Cardiology
Dermatology	Palliative Medicine
Endocrinology and Diabetes Mellitus	Pharmaceutical Medicine
Gastroenterology	Rehabilitation Medicine
General (Internal) Medicine	Renal Medicine
Genitourinary Medicine	Respiratory Medicine
Geriatric Medicine	Rheumatology
Haematology	Sport and Exercise Medicine
Immunology	Stroke Medicine

Physician Training Pathway

During the F2 year physicians must apply for two years of Core Medical Training (CMT1-2), which is designed to give a core grounding in general medicine.

Following successful completion of the Core Medical Training years medics may then apply for medical registrar jobs in either general medicine or in a specialist field.

Postgraduate Examinations

The Royal College of Physicians oversees postgraduate training for medics. The Membership of the Royal College of Physicians (MRCP) consists of three parts and may be started during the F2 year. The MRCP is challenging due to the quantity of knowledge required of the medical syllabus.

MRCP Part I Multiple choice question paper assessing basic science knowledge

MRCP Part II Extended matching questions with focus on your clinical knowledge

MRCP Part III (also called PACES) This assesses practical clinical skills and interpretation using an objective structured clinical examination (OSCE) format which is similar to MMI stations.

Key Points

- Physicians diagnose and treat medical conditions

- Applied medical knowledge and deductive skills are required

- Medical on calls are usually very busy

- Medical patients form the majority of hospital inpatients

- Medical training is not as competitive as Surgery or GP

BEING A SURGEON

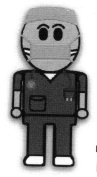

Surgeons are able to quickly identify life or limb-threatening problems and immediately treat conditions with operative procedures. Surgeons must not only possess a high level of medical knowledge they must also be adept with practical skills and calm under pressure.

The word surgery is derived from the Greek term 'cheiros' meaning 'hand' and it is desirable for a surgeon to possess both manual dexterity and spatial awareness.

What Surgeons Do

Surgery is a craft and historically surgeons were trained as apprentices while living and working under a master surgeon. Today surgeons work on hospital wards, in clinics and in operating departments. Surgeons have the privilege of being able to quickly improve the condition of a patient by performing an operation.

> **Example (General Surgery):** A 22-year-old male dentist is admitted to the surgical assessment unit (SAU) after visiting his GP with right iliac fossa (right lower abdomen) pain for the last 12 hours that is getting worse. His blood inflammatory markers are high, he has a temperature and the surgeons examine his abdomen and decide he has appendicitis. He is taken to theatre for a laparoscopic (key hole) appendicectomy. His inflamed appendix is removed and he leaves hospital the following day.

A surgical day usually begins early (before 8am) with a trauma meeting or ward round. Here the surgical patients admitted during the previous 24 hours are discussed and reviewed by the surgical Consultant on call. A surgical 'firm' is composed of a Consultant, a Registrar, a Core Surgical

Trainee and one or two Foundation Doctors. The Foundation Doctors are responsible for looking after the ward patients and completing tasks from the ward round while the more senior team members attend clinic and theatre.

Surgery is fast paced with all-day theatre lists beginning at 9am (hence the early 8am start). In theatre consultants teach Registrars, Core Trainees and F1/2s how to perform operations and trainees often come in on their days off to make sure their surgical skills are up to scratch (operating is also lots of fun). Theatre staff play an important role in ensuring that equipment is clean and patients are ready for theatre and surgery is very much a team-based specialty.

Teaching and research are particularly important in surgery and surgeons are expected to teach peers and undertake projects on designated research days and in their own time. Most research culminates with a publication in a surgical journal or presentation at a conference.

Surgical Specialties

Surgery covers ten distinct surgical specialties each of which is further divided into subspecialties:

General Surgery: abdomen, breast and thyroid	**ENT:** Ear nose and throat
Trauma and Orthopaedic Surgery: fractures, joints and limb injuries	**Paediatric Surgery:** children's surgery
Neurosurgery: skull and brain	**Maxillofacial Surgery:** facial and dental injuries
Plastic Surgery: burns and soft-tissue reconstruction	**Cardiothoracic Surgery:** hearts and lungs
Urology: the urinary tract	**Vascular Surgery:** blood vessels

Each specialty is further divided into its own subspecialties. For example, general surgery can be broken down into breast surgery, colorectal (the large bowel, rectum and anus) surgery, upper gastrointestinal (liver and gall bladder) surgery and endocrine surgery.

Surgical Training Pathway

The training pathway for surgeons is long and arduous but being able to transform people's lives and work in private practice justifies the hard work.

Application to Core Surgical Training (CT1-2) takes place during the F2 year. The application process is competitive and only the top candidates are chosen after interview. During the CT years surgeons may spend their four six month placements in general surgery or any of the other surgical specialties.

During the CT2 year applications open for Registrar (ST3) posts. Each surgical specialty has their own training programme so trainees wanting to become plastic surgeons apply to the plastics ST3 programme while those wanting to be orthopaedic surgeons apply to the orthopaedic programme.

Registrar training lasts for six years and trainees may then apply for consultant posts.

Postgraduate Courses and Exams

Surgical training is expensive. To apply for Registrar posts trainees must have passed Basic Surgical Skills (BSS), Advanced Trauma and Life Support (ATLS) and Care of the Critically Ill Surgical Patient (CRISP) courses. They must also have passed both parts of the Membership of The Royal College of Surgeons (MRCS) and Fellowship of the Royal College of Surgeons (FRCS) Exams. Each of these costs around £500 and trainees are expected to pay for these themselves.

During surgical training there are two major exams. The MRCS a two-part exam, taken during the Foundation or Core Training period.

MRCS Part A Four-hour multiple-choice examination, which tests knowledge of the applied sciences of medicine and clinical problem solving.

A comprehensive knowledge of anatomy, physiology and pathology and their application in the real world is needed.

MRCS Part B An Objective Structured Clinical Examination (OSCE) consisting of 16 stations where the candidate has the opportunity to demonstrate their competence as a surgeon.

Once these two exams are passed the candidate may change his or her title back to Mr or Miss, harking back to the tradition of Barber surgeons being called Mr and not Dr.

Towards the end of specialty training an exit exam, the FRCS (Fellowship of the Royal College of Surgeons), is taken.

Key Points

- Surgery requires dexterity and strong practical skills

- Surgical training is long, taking around ten years to reach consultant level

- There are lots of mandatory exams and courses that trainees must fund themselves

- Competition for posts is fierce with only the best selected

BEING A GENERAL PRACTITIONER (GP)

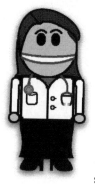

General Practitioners are the gatekeepers to the NHS. Most people visit their local GP at some stage in their lives and you may already have a good understanding of what a GP's role is within the UK healthcare system.

The vast majority of medical school graduates will go on to become GPs and the escape from the on calls and stresses of hospital medicine can be very appealing to some.

What General Practitioners Do

GPs work together in GP 'practices' or 'surgeries'. A practice/surgery is made up of a number of GP partners who, like hospital consultants, have finished their training. Foundation doctors on GP placements and GP trainees will also work at the practice as will nurses, physios and pharmacists.

GPs usually begin their day between 8-9am. Their day is divided into clinic appointments at the practice and home visits to patients who are unable to visit the practice. GPs will often have time set aside for speaking with patients over the phone (phone triage) and for teaching trainees.

GPs have around 7 minutes in which to see patients in their clinics, reach a diagnosis and offer treatment advice. Patients attend GP surgeries with a vast array of problems from pregnant mothers to depressed teenagers to painful knees to newborn babies. GPs are required to have a very generalist knowledge of medicine and can refer specific cases to the appropriate hospital specialty if they require further advice. This variety in both presenting complaints and the characters that you meet is very appealing for those who enjoy talking with people and thinking quickly.

Though generalists at heart GPs can choose to specialise in a certain area. This might be sports medicine, dermatology, obstetrics or emergency medicine. This allows GPs to focus their interest and remain skilled in a specific area.

Along with their medical role GPs also have a strong management role having been put in charge of local funding budgets. Most GP practices have managers and are run using a business model. Practices may incorporate their own pharmacy into their building, employ additional nurses or physios to run clinics or offer private medicals for travel or work.

GP Training Pathway

Becoming a GP is appealing as GP training is the shortest in all of medicine. Due to its short length many budding GPs take a year out after F2 to work abroad in countries such as Australia or New Zealand.

The GP application opens in the foundation year 2 year. Unlike other speciality applications, there is less emphasis on publications, audits, courses or experience. Instead GP applicants are required to take a two-part multiple-choice exam. This is devised to test both the general medical knowledge of the candidate as well as their decision-making and prioritising abilities.

Following the exam there is a station-based assessment. The first station involves a written task prioritising a number of problems, justifying your reasons and reflecting on the process. The next three stations are simulations with actors playing a patient, a relative and another healthcare professional assessing your communication skills, empathy, and decision making.

GP training lasts three years after Foundation year two. The first two years of GP training focus on hospital medicine rotating around specialties such as obstetrics and gynaecology, old age medicine, trauma and orthopaedics and paediatrics. The third year is spent in a GP practice.

After completion of specialist training you are now a GP. From here the aim is usually to become a principal or partner of a surgery. However, opportunities for this are limited, and it may take some years working as a salaried-GP, building a relationship with a practice, and waiting for an opportunity to arise before this happens.

Postgraduate Examinations

In their second or third year of GP training, trainees are required to complete their MRCGP (Membership of the Royal College of General Practitioners). The exam is composed of two parts:

Applied Knowledge Test (AKT) A multiple choice exam covering generalist medical topics.

Clinical Skills Assessment (CSA) A practical "simulated" type exam. In addition to this, trainees must complete a computer based e-portfolio of work based assessments, and their own reflections.

Key Points

• General Practitioners require a broad medical knowledge

• GP training is the shortest in medicine lasting just three years

• GPs are involved in healthcare funding at local and regional levels

• Communication and empathy are key skills

• The short training time offers opportunities to work abroad, as a locum and to pursue other interests

BEING AN ANAESTHETIST

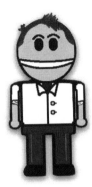

Anaesthetists or 'anaesthesiologists', as they are known in the United States, are often thought of as the doctors who 'put patients to sleep for surgery'. While this is a large part of anaesthetics, anaesthetists are highly specialised medical doctors who deal with many of the sickest patients in the hospital. Anaesthetists provide care and emergency resuscitation to critically ill patients in hospital Intensive Care Units (ITUs) and in emergency situations.

What Anaesthetists Do

Anaesthetists are the largest group of doctors in the hospital and their expert skills in airway and breathing management are widely used in patient care. While much of an anaesthetist's time is spent ensuring patients are adequately anaesthetised for surgical operations anaesthetists are also involved in the optimisation of patients for surgery, the relief of postoperative pain, in managing cardiac or respiratory arrests, running intensive care units and assisting with chronic pain management.

Anaesthetists usually start their day with the surgeons (before 8am) and will start their day by seeing the patients on the day's operating list to ensure they are fit for surgery. The anaesthetist and their trainee will decide upon the type of anaesthetic to use, the requirement for postoperative pain relief and any other factors that might complicate the operation. Once they are happy they will liaise with the surgeon and wait for the first patient to be brought to the operating department.

Anaesthetists use their practical skills to administer a general or spinal anaesthetic to the patient and then monitor their physiological parameters while the patient is asleep before bringing the patient round at the end of the procedure.

Though operating lists takes up the majority of their time anaesthetists may choose to train down the acute anaesthetics training pathway and become ITU consultants using their expert medical knowledge to look after the sickest patients in the hospital.

Indeed, the majority of consultant anaesthetists will have a sub-speciality or special area of interest. These might include: paediatric, cardiac, cardiothoracic, ENT, pain management, trauma, obstetrics and neurosurgery.

When on call anaesthetists will be the first to crash calls and emergencies and are responsible for stabilising a patient's airway before deciding whether they need admission to an intensive care setting. In this respect the job can be exciting but also stressful.

Due to the large volume of anaesthetists required to staff ITUs and operating lists trainees gain a one-to-one teaching experience from consultant anaesthetists during their training.

Anaesthetic Training Pathway

The Royal College of Anaesthetists (RCOA) governs the postgraduate anaesthetic training pathway.

Application to Core Anaesthetic Training (CT1-2) years takes place during Foundation Year 2.

CT1-2 years are focused on the trainee developing their basic competencies at anaesthetics. It begins with a three-month period where the trainee must rapidly develop their experience, knowledge and understanding of anaesthetics and be shown to be competent to a specific criteria of knowledge and ability. After these 3 months the trainee is then allowed to work on the on call rota under close supervision delivering anaesthetics to emergency surgical patients. At this stage this usually doesn't entail night shifts. Along with their on call responsibilities they rotate through a core set of specialities, and must show to develop competencies in each. After a while it is usual for the trainee to take responsibilities on the obstetric on call rota with slightly more distant supervision, often working at night.

Postgraduate Exams

Anaesthetists must pass two examinations before they become consultants. Trainees are required to sit the Primary RCOA Fellowship Exam before becoming a registrar. The exam is in two separate parts:

Part A A multiple choice exam with single best answer questions.

Part B Is OSCE and viva based. The exam tests trainees' knowledge of anatomy, physics, pharmacology, biochemistry and physiology.

Trainees are expected to pass the Final Fellowship Examination during their Intermediate level of training (CT3-4). The Syllabus is a lot more 'applied' than the Primary exam and tests the trainees knowledge that they have built on from the Primary in a clinical setting. This is in two parts with a written part, and a viva style part.

Key Points

- Anaesthetists are the largest group of doctors in the hospital

- Anaesthetists put patients to sleep for operations but also use their skills in airway management to manage some of the sickest patients in the hospital

- Training is long but there is good support from consultants

- Training can be flexible with options to take time out of training to pursue other interests When To Start Preparing

Chapter 3: Work Experience

Undertaking work experience in a hospital, GP surgery or volunteering will give you a feel for what life as a doctor entails. It will ensure that you are making the right career choice and will increase your chances of performing well at medical school interviews.

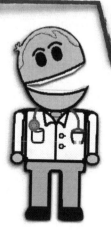

WHEN AND HOW MUCH?

Experiencing working life is a vital component of choosing any career and succeeding at university interviews. While you may have preconceived ideas about what life is like as a doctor from second hand experiences through family, friends or the media there is no substitute for experiencing what doctors do on a daily basis. Medicine is not just about attaining A-Level grades and university interview panels will want to know that you are aware of what training to be a doctor and working as a doctor entails and that you have evidence of voluntary work demonstrating empathy.

By undertaking work experience you will be able to ensure that medicine is the career for you and learn the difficulties and daily tasks facing doctors to give a balanced account of your experiences at interview.

We recommend approaching any work experience in structured, stepwise manner:

Plan, Organise, Prepare, Attend, Reflect

When to Do Work Experience

As mentioned above work experience is valuable for two main reasons:

- **To ensure medicine is the career for you**
- **To gain experiences and insights that can be utilised at interview**

If you are unsure about medical school we recommend organising work experience in medicine together with other careers to give you a good idea of what you may wish to do.

As suggested in Chapter 1 work experience is best organised for during Year 11 or after GCSE exams. Most hospitals, courses and organisations are happy to have Year 11 students undertaking work experiences with them.

Getting started early is key as organising placements, jobs or booking experience days can take time and you want to do your homework to ensure the experiences are the best they can be.

We would suggest you start thinking about things before Christmas time of Year 11, if you have received this book as a Christmas present you are in good standing!

You may then wish to gain further experience during Year 12 before interviews. Voluntary work is best undertaken as an ongoing experience over a number of months or years and this can be started as early as Year 10.

Due to the fast-paced nature of medicine and the need to protect patient confidentiality and safety it can be difficult for school students to organise solid medical work experience. Many students with no connections to medicine also have no idea about how to go about organising work placements. Luckily there are plenty of opportunities to gain enjoyable and rewarding medical experiences if you know where to look.

How Much Work Experience?

The simple answer to this is 'the more the better'. The reality is that you will have other commitments such as schoolwork, extracurricular and social activities that will take up much of your time and doing lengthily shadowing placements is not always necessary. Most students gain these by doing two or three weeks of work experience placements and longer, on going volunteering or part-time work together with attending medical experience courses to give a solid summary of medicine.

On the next page you will find our suggested work experience.

Suggested Work Experience

Hospital Work Experience: 2 weeks covering a variety of specialties

GP Work Experience: 72hrs to 1 week

Voluntary: On going volunteering at a hospice, care home or other for around 1 morning or after school per week for 4-12 months

Experience Courses: Attend an experience day to give you an idea of life as a doctor, the different career paths, medical school and the application process.

Insider's Edge 5

"I organised hospital work experience through a family friend who was a respiratory consultant. I spent two weeks shadowing the F1 doctors on the wards and saw patients in clinics. The team were really helpful and organised for me to spend time in other departments such as A&E, cardiology and general surgery. I saw how the F1s are the first point of contact for the nursing staff and spend much of their time completing paper work to meet hospital targets. After this placement I organised a week in a bariatric surgery unit as this was something I was interested in and the interviewers were interested to hear what I had learned about obesity and how bariatric surgery works."

PLANNING WORK EXPERIENCE

While shadowing a junior doctor in a hospital and volunteering at a care home or hospice are well-known forms of medical work experience there are a number of options available to you. Although it is not necessary to gain experience from all the methods below doing something different or extra will often make you stand out from the hundreds of other applicants at interview.

Hospital Specialties

There are a number of hospital-based specialties looking after different types of patients and performing vastly different daily activities. For example surgeons will be operating in theatre, holding clinics or admitting elective or emergency cases while physicians will be doing lengthily ward rounds, holding multidisciplinary meetings and assessing unwell medical patients. While it is not necessary to shadow every hospital-based specialty it is useful to spend some of your work experience appreciating the differences between specialties including what types of patients they look after and what the junior doctors are required to do.

Our basic suggestion is to spend a week in a medical placement and a week in a surgical placement with a few days or afternoons spent observing specific specialties such as radiology, microbiology, pathology, bariatric surgery or anything else.

Below are some specific specialties that you may be interested in shadowing:

Cardiology There will be lots to see and do from the normal shadowing of juniors to attending pacing clinic, learning about how drugs affect the heart and seeing ECHOs performed.

Respiratory Patients with respiratory infections, COPD, asthma or lung cancers are cared for on respiratory wards. You may get to practise assessing breathing using peak flow meters, see BIPAP used to help patients breathe and learn about infectious diseases.

Neurology You will be able to learn about how MRI and CT scans can image the brain, see how neurological disease can be debilitating and observe lumbar punctures and electroencephalography (EEG) being performed.

Old Age Medicine This encompasses much of general medicine with elderly patients having many co-morbidities. Work experience offers a great opportunity to see the 'bread-and-butter' of medicine and to appreciate difficulties facing the elderly population.

General Surgery General surgeons operate on elective and emergency cases and cover abdominal conditions such as appendicitis, hernias or gallstones. General surgery work experience placements allow you to see patients on the wards, in clinic and in theatre.

Trauma & Orthopaedic Surgery Orthopaedic surgeons operate on broken bones and help patients with painful joints or fractures. Work experience is great as there are opportunities to shadow ward doctors, attend clinics, attend trauma meetings and if you are lucky see an operation.

Radiology Radiologists look at X-ray, CT, MRI and USS images and report them. They also perform interventional procedures under image guidance. You will see patients having scans but there are no junior doctors and it is probably better to spend an afternoon in the department rather than a whole week.

Anaesthetics Anaesthetists are based in theatres or ITU and as such it may be difficult to access work experience with them. If you can go to theatre or ITU anaesthetics will give you an excellent account of patient experiences and critically unwell patients.

Microbiology Microbiologists tend to do a long ward-round of all hospitals patients with severe infections or on specialised antibiotics. Microbiology work experience is outside the norm and helps you to stand out and learning about antibiotics and bugs gives you something specific to talk about at interview.

General Practice

General practice is very different from the fast-paced setting of a hospital. Work experience at a GP surgery will allow you to see plenty of different illnesses and go on home visits with the GP. It is important that you appreciate the role of GPs and the differences to hospital specialties. You might also be able to talk to trainees about their training programme and learn about the managerial and financial sides of running a practice.

Volunteering

Volunteering and demonstrating empathy and a desire to help others is a mandatory part of the medical school application process. As described later on in the interview chapter, medical school interviewers are looking for evidence of on going volunteering and not just a day or a week.

There are many ways to volunteer and show your caring side. Try to pick something that you will enjoy as no voluntary job is better than another. Below are a few popular suggestions:

Care or Residential Home Sometimes elderly people find it a struggle to look after themselves and manage at home. Care homes provide a safe environment for elderly patients to live and be in the company of others. As a volunteer you can talk to the residents, help make tea or help the staff clean and organise their days.

Nursing Home Diseases such as dementia or neurological conditions mean that people may be unable to do even basic things for themselves such as washing, dressing or eating. Nursing homes are run by trained nurses able to offer complete care to patients. Your role may be to help feed or wash patients and tends to be more hands-on than care homes.

Hospice Patients with terminal disease often require specialist end-of-life care and hospices provide safe environments that allow family members to visit. Work experience here will give you a valuable insight into how medicine can care for patients with terminal conditions and how staff, patients and families cope with death.

Hospital Most hospitals have volunteers who help staff shops, deliver mail to departments and read to patients on wards. Volunteering in hospitals has the added bonus of more easily being able to access routes into hospital work experience and will allow you to see hospital-based care.

Carers Sometimes people with disabilities or elderly patients still living at home benefit from care at home. You can often help by simply talking with people who may be lonely living by themselves.

Local Support Group Local venues often run groups for elderly patients or patients with a certain illness to meet and share stories. You could help meet people, make tea and learn about the difficulties they face.

Special Needs Group There are a number of opportunities available to help people with special needs from helping with swimming lessons for the disabled to talking to people with special needs at a local club.

Charity Work While there is limited exposure to patients raising money for charity through sport, events or challenges demonstrates both a caring attitude and the ability to complete a demanding task. Raising money looks great on any CV and is best done in addition to one of the above voluntary jobs.

Youth Work While not as easily relatable to medicine as the above helping at local scouts or brownies and youth centres is another way to demonstrate caring and develop leadership and teamwork skills.

Research and Audit

Research and audit are key components of the NHS. Research is somewhat of an abstract term and is essentially about obtaining new knowledge and finding out what treatments are the most effective. Audit in contrast assess whether current practices are meeting set standards. Essentially research attempts to define and identify best standards for care while audit ensures that standards are being maintained.

Doctors often take time out of clinical practice to undertake research within their chosen field and professors run research departments funded by the government to advance medical knowledge.

Audits in contrast are ongoing within every hospital department and involve all doctors.

Work experience in a research department is not particularly common but will give you a fantastic understanding of a different side of medicine and you may even be able to play a role in a project yourself. Becoming involved in an audit will also help you to understand this side of medicine.

Experience Days and Courses

Even the most well organised hospital placements may not give you a complete overview of a career in medicine. Medical experience days give you a focussed, broad insight into life in medicine and are a valuable adjunct to work experience. Courses will help you show commitment to medicine together with offering insights into the application process.

Selecting the right course can be tricky and it is recommended that you ensure the course is run by people with insight into the medical school application process. Hospitals often run courses and lectures for school leavers and there are lots of courses run locally or nationally that you can attend.

The Royal Society of Medicine Some national medical organisations such as the RSM run lectures aimed at school students and lay-people on interesting medical topics and careers.

The Royal College of Surgeons The RCSEng and RCSEd run workshops and tours of their museums for school students. Doctors are on hand to show you suturing and videos of surgical procedures and it is usually good fun. Visiting one of the medical museums also gives you something to show commitment at interview.

The Royal College of Physicians The college of physicians runs a dedicated day for prospective medical students similar to the above.

Skills Courses

Having gained work experience and attended a medical experience day skills courses are a great way to augment your application and make you stand out. Skills courses include life support courses and medical and surgical skills days that will help you at interview and in the future.

First Aid and Life Support Local hospitals and community centres often run introductory courses to give you an idea of how to help people with basic injuries. St John's Ambulance and Red Cross websites also offer a range of courses nationwide.

Medsim Based in Nottingham this course is held over a week and gives you an idea of life as a university student. There is a strong commercial focus with private universities from Europe featuring heavily and it is important to be wary of this.

Paid Work Experience

In the current financial climate getting paid and gaining experience in a medical setting is very sensible. Medical work is often shift-based and can involve night shifts. For this reason it is best undertaken at weekends or during summer holidays and it is important that it does not interfere with your schoolwork. Jobs can be organised by contacting your local hospital

HR department or through the NHS jobs website. There is often a waiting list for shifts during the summer and it is best to sign up early to so that you are added to the staff bank. No prior experience is required and there is usually an induction period.

Health Care Assistant Shifts pay £6-8 per hour and involve assisting nurses on the wards. Tasks may include recording blood pressures, washing patients, helping patients to the bathroom and changing beds. Shifts are usually 8 hours.

Portering Porters move patients, notes and equipment around the hospital. Pay is around £5-7 per hour and is shift-based.

Allied Healthcare Professionals

It is important that you appreciate the roles of other healthcare professionals in the work place as you will be working closely with them during your future career. Understanding how their roles differ from doctors is also important when answering common interview questions such as 'why be a doctor rather than a nurse/physio?'. It is not necessary to spend an entire week with allied healthcare professionals but an afternoon of shadowing during your hospital work placement can be eye-opening.

Nurses Nursing staff look after patients on the ward. They are often short-staffed and their jobs require patience and knowledge of when to seek help from doctors.

Physios Helping to rehabilitate patients prior to discharge from hospital is vitally important. Physios work with patients to improve their mobility and ability to function independently.

Paramedics Going out with paramedics is great fun and looks equally good on your application. Due to health and safety restrictions it is not as easy to gain work experience as it once was but there is certainly no harm in enquiring through your local hospital or St John's Ambulance.

Going Abroad

If you want to do something amazing, have the money and enjoy travelling companies such as GapMedics can help to organise gap year or vacation placements in hospitals in countries such as Tanzania, China and Argentina. This requires a level of maturity and independence and is certainly not necessary but offers some exciting experiences to talk about at interview and a viable way to add to your application if you are not offered a place first time around.

Special Interests and Unique Placements

Together with the above suggestions there are a multitude of other specialised medical experiences that you could add to your armoury. Local hospitals may run specific courses or days for students or there may be a specialised unit with a unique treatment close to where you live. These can usually be sampled in a 1-2 day placement and adds something extra to your application.

Below are a few examples of unique placements that have stood out in recent medical school interviews and applications. All the below examples are unique and we encourage you to be creative and make yourself stand out from the crowd. Whatever it is you choose remember that interviewers are looking for specific examples and what you have learned from them at interview.

Hyperbaric Unit These are used to treat divers with 'the bends' and have also been used to promote healing in burn injuries. The student in question went on a day when there was a lecture to junior doctors about the unit and was able to ask them questions also.

Stimulation Suite The Bristol Royal Infirmary allows work experience students to use their world-class simulation suite, which features a robotic mannequin to simulate how to treat unwell patients. This is a fantastic opportunity to understand both clinical medicine and modern teaching tools used to train doctors.

Sports Medicine GPs often have a specialist interest in sports medicine and act as medical cover for local sporting events or as team doctors for football or rugby clubs. One student had arranged to shadow a GP at a rugby match and saw him relocate a dislocated finger and a shoulder.

Events Medicine Doctors often cover events such as motor sports, horse racing and marathons and triathlons. The doctors deal with any injuries to competitors or spectators and can vary from having no work all day to a major trauma injury. One student had followed a team at a local Indy car-racing event for a day organising it through a consultant he had met while in a hospital placement.

ORGANISING WORK EXPERIENCE

For students with no access to medicine through family or friends it can seem very intimidating to even know where to start when it comes to organising medical work experience. Indeed even for students with family members or friends who are medics choices may be limited to the hospital or department that they work in.

Clinical Work Experience (Hospital and GP)

Different hospitals and GP practices will have different policies on work experience. Some will helpfully organise programmes for local schools while other may limit the number of work experience placements. It is important to search for placements at all the hospitals in your area and not settle for closest one. Most work experience placements require a criminal record check and a school reference (as a paid job does) and you should factor in potential delays as they can take time to process.

It is important to note that some hospitals have set policies on where you can and can't visit for work experience for example some hospitals want students to be at least 17 to attend Paediatrics and it can be difficult to enter theatres without the direct permission of the supervising consultant if you are under 18.

Below are tried and tested methods of organising work experience:

Family and Friends The first and easiest place to begin is utilising family members or family friends who are doctors or have links to medical professionals. If you know the person well, expressing an interest and telling them how long you wish to spend in a specific placement is usually enough.

If you are given a contact or you do not know the person well the best policy is to send them a polite email expressing an interest. Being specific shows that you have done your homework and will help the person tailor the placement to your needs.

"Dear Mr Bone,

I was given your secretary's email address by Mr James Foot, a family friend, who indicated that you might be able to help me organise a work experience placement in your department.

I am currently in Year 11 (GCSE year) and would ideally like to spend two weeks in July in the hospital shadowing the junior doctors, attending clinic, attending the trauma meeting and seeing patients before and after operations. I would also like to spend time in a medical specialty to get a balanced view of what medicine entails.

Any help that you could offer would be very much appreciated.

Kind regards,"

It is important to remember that doctors are busy and they might not get back to you immediately or may not be the correct person to help. If you do not receive the desired reply do not be disheartened and simply try again. If someone doesn't get back to you within a week don't be afraid to chase them up. Be relentless.

Medical Students Leavers from your school who have gone on to medical school are another good source of tips and contacts. If you weren't close friends with them teachers may be able to help you get in touch.

Asking at School Some schools have hospital contacts or have sent students on specific programmes and can point you in the right direction. This is not always the case and sometimes more detective work is needed.

Hospital Programmes Some hospitals run specific work experience programmes for school students. These can usually be found on the hospital's website under the 'work for us' sub page. If it is not obvious searching the website for 'work experience' can yield hidden pages.

Hospital HR Departments If the hospital website does not mention a work experience programme it is still worth checking the hospital human resources department to ensure that there isn't one. HR departments can be contacted through hospital websites or through the hospital switchboard.

Consultant's Secretaries If you do not know anyone who has direct access to medical work experience it is up to you to make contact with the hospital yourself.

Top Tip

Most hospital websites have sub-pages listing doctors who work in each department. These sub-pages often have email addresses or telephone numbers for the secretaries of consultants. You can then send an email enquiring about work experience. If there is only a telephone number you should phone the secretary and ask about work experience or for an email address to put the request in writing. If there are no contact details on the website you can phone the hospital switchboard directly and ask to be put through to one of the consultant's secretaries or you could google the consultant to see if they have an alternative contact address.

Networking One of the advantages of attending medical experience days or doing paid work in a hospital is that it offers you a chance to ask doctors about work experience. It is also important to network during placements themselves as you may hear about another exciting opportunity to shadow a different department or a unique opportunity such as those mentioned above.

GP Surgeries You may know your GP well if you have had to visit them in the past and they will be well-positioned to help you organise work experience at their practice or suggest who the best person to contact at the local hospital is. You should ring or email the GP surgery to enquire about work experience and most will be very accommodating.

Medical Schools If you are still struggling a good option is to go to the website of your local university medical school and look for a contact for the undergraduate or admissions office. Medical schools send students to hospitals and GP practices all around the region and they will have contacts that should be able to help.

Volunteering

Undertaking voluntary work experience is a little more straightforward to organise as most hospices, care homes or support groups will be glad of the help. If you know a local hospice, care home or community centre that is easy for you to regularly attend either at weekends or for a day after school then they should be your first port of call. It is vital that you choose a voluntary job that you will both enjoy and that you can easily visit. If you are still unsure a great place to start are charity, volunteering or local council websites which offer information on types of volunteering together with locations of facilities. Below are some practical suggestions to help you organise the best voluntary work experience possible.

Family and Friends As above the best starting point is to ask people you know whether this is family, school leavers or teachers at school. Some may be involved in community work and know contacts at local facilities.

Local Hospice or Care Home You may well already know a hospice or care home in your area. If so they may have a website with volunteering opportunities or you could drop in or phone up to enquire about helping.

Duke of Edinburgh Scheme Most students undertake the D of E and it is a great way to develop leadership and teamwork skills. The programme involves you in community activities and requires upwards of 18months of volunteering for the gold award, which nicely fits in with your medical school volunteering needs. The D of E website also has a search function for locating volunteering opportunities in your area.

Community Centres Many local community centres run specific services for patients. This might include a physio-led balance workshop for the elderly, meetings for patients with disabilities or breaks for carers. A quick web search of the local community centres in your area will often reveal lots of opportunities on their website. You could also raise money for your local community centre and some centres run first aid courses making these a great source of value.

Local Council Website These will have links to websites for community centres, volunteer centres and to other volunteering and community opportunities in your area.

Volunteering Websites Sites such as www.volunteering.org.uk and www.do-it.org.uk offer contact details for a number of volunteering opportunities by region and give a good overview of other ways you can help your community.

Charities The Red Cross, Sue Ryder. Mencap and many other charities recruit volunteers through their websites. They have a variety of volunteering opportunities at local and national level and will be able to put you in contact with homes, hospices and groups in your area.

MAKING THE MOST OF WORK EXPERIENCE

Depending on how you have organised your work experience you should be sent a date, timetable and any other paperwork or information that is required o be completed.

Ensure that you get any required paperwork back to the necessary people in good time as delays could affect your placement. If there is anything you are not sure about in the timetable or that you would like to change it is worth emailing the lead organiser early to get changes implemented before you start.

It is sensible to write down questions that you might like answered. There are no stupid questions and doctors will expect you to know nothing and ask lots. Questions should cover anything you are unsure about or find interesting or important and you can even ask about medical applications and opportunities for further work experience. We advise being dynamic and showing interest to get the most information out of doctors.

Below are some tools and suggestions to help you get the most out of your work experiences:

What to Wear and What to Take

Most placements will inform you of the required dress code but if they do not always ask if you are unsure.

For men polished shoes, smart trousers and belt and a plain, ironed shirt are a necessity. Most wards operate a bare below the elbows policy so sleeves should be rolled up and watch removed. Hospitals have different policies on ties, we recommend wearing one but tucking it into your shirt and only removing it if asked.

For women smart shoes and skirt and plain jumper or shirt will be fine.

It is worth taking a bag with a pen and small pad to take notes, printed copy of directions and timetable and lunch and some spare cash.

Most doctors carry phones in their pockets and, due to the use of medical apps, wards are relaxed about their use. It is important that you wear an identification badge which should be provided by before or on your first day of work.

What to get from Your Time

This is looked at in detail in the reflection section below but it is important to mention that if this is your first experience of healthcare your primary goal is to understand the roles of healthcare professionals, what their job entails, how their actions affect patients and the difficulties they face in their working lives and in balancing their time outside of work. You will pick up bits of information about diseases and treatment options and this can be explored in greater detail in your own time or in a further placement. Your goals are to get a feel for life as a doctor and ensure that you can picture yourself doing this job in the future.

A Typical Day in Hospital

Most hospital-based placements begin with a ward round of the current inpatients. Depending on the specialty this can be quick (surgery) or very long (medicine). The ward round will be led by a consultant or one of the junior doctors and it can be an overload of information and sights for anyone new to the environment. For the first ward round it is best to observe what the doctors do, where the notes are kept, what they look at on the observation and drug charts and how the doctors interact with the patients.

During the ward round the foundation doctor will have written down jobs on his or her patient list as they arose. Following the ward round they will prioritise these tasks, undertaking the most important ones first. Jobs will vary depending on the specialty but they usually involve requesting tests, contacting other teams, taking blood or writing a discharge summary.

Lunch will either be in the canteen or in the doctor's mess. It is advisable to take your own lunch as many doctors do this and canteen food may not be to your liking.

You will either spend the rest of the day shadowing or observing senior doctors in specialty clinics. Clinics are a great way to see a variety of patients and doctors will see both new patients referred by GPs for specialist assessment and follow up patients who are under observation.

The day normally finishes at 5pm and you shouldn't have to stay longer than this.

A Guide to Being a Hospital Shadow

The term 'shadowing' refers to you following around a doctor or healthcare professional as if you were their shadow. However your work experience is timetabled a significant portion will involve shadowing as this gives you the greatest exposure to life in medicine. The key to both enjoying and being a good work experience student is to interact with the team and ask questions. Some doctors may prefer you not to help with tasks but it is worth offering to get or put away notes as the thought will be appreciated.

Make sure that you know the grade of the doctor you are shadowing and how long they have worked in the job to relate what they do to their level of experience.

Taking notes and observing everything that goes on is also important, as you will almost certainly forget things after a busy day.

It is important to understand that doctors are busy and their first priority is to look after the patients and complete jobs before they go home so do not be offended if you are not their main focus. Instead see it as an opportunity to watch them work and see how they deal with challenges.

While shadowing on the ward round or on call you may be overloaded with information about why patients are in hospital or the drugs they are taking, try to take some notes that you can then ask about later or look up when you get home.

Walking between wards to see patients is a good opportunity to strike up conversation with the team and get to know them. Simple questions such as how long have you worked here? Do you live locally? Which medical school did you go to? Together with the questions below will be appreciated and make you appear less awkward.

Finally make sure that together with shadowing doctors you also observe or shadow a nurse or a physio for a few hours to get an idea of what their job entails and how it differs from that of a doctor.

A Guide to Being a GP Surgery Shadow

GPs will have more time to answer your questions and it is important to utilise their generalist knowledge. Some patients will not want a student to sit in on their consultations but most will be happy to help with your future training. GP surgeries usually open at 0830 and consultations take place in the GP's room lasting around seven minutes. The GP may take phone calls or visit patients in their home.

Most surgeries will have nurse-led clinics such as contraceptive advice, dressing clinics, wound clinics or blood tests.

GPs may have a specialist interest in a particular area and you might get a chance to see things like minor surgery, immunisation clinics or alternative medicines.

There will be foundation doctors and GP trainees working at the surgery too together with nurses and receptionists and they can prove a valuable source of information.

Questions to Ask

Work experience is a fantastic opportunity to ask as many questions as possible. Many students are overwhelmed by being in a hospital and do not know what to ask. A good frame to come from is to imagine yourself as an interviewer or documentary maker who will not want to cause a disruption but who wants to capture all the action and ask the important questions. Below are some helpful suggestions, which should prepare you for the interview section later. Remember you should ask questions of everyone not just doctors.

Questions For Doctors

What is the rota like?

How often are you on call and how often do you work nights and weekends?

What is the best/worst thing about the job?

What was the best/worst thing about medical school?

Knowing what you know now would you still do medicine or a different career?

Where do you live? What is hospital accommodation like?

What is your most memorable experience?

How much do you earn a month?

What car do you drive?

What did you do to get into medical school? Can you offer any advice?

Can you suggest any extra work experience/courses/volunteering?

Are there any opportunities to get involved with an audit/research?

Can you suggest a good answer to this interview question…?

Which of your friends enjoys their job the most?

Questions For Patients

What brought you into hospital?

What has the hospital experience been like for you so far?

Have you been in hospital before?

What did you do for work?

What is the worst thing about being in hospital?

Do you understand what is currently happening?

Questions For Nurses

What makes a good doctor?

What is the hardest part of your job?

How long are your shifts?

Did you always want to be a nurse?

Why did you choose nursing?

What have been the biggest changes since you qualified?

What I Wish I'd Known

Below are a few things that students and doctors wished they had known before attending work experience:

" Foundation doctors are often scared themselves when dealing with unwell patients or when asked to do something outside of their comfort zone. "

"Discharge summaries are the bane of most foundation doctors' lives. They are meant to be a way for information about the patient's admission to be quickly sent to the GP but in reality are time consuming and take doctors away from patient-centred jobs."

" Imaging such as X-rays, CTs, MRIs and USS must be requested. This involves the doctor filling out a form and delivering it to the radiology department."

" Doctors don't know every drug. They learn common prescriptions at medical school and on the job and for everything else they look up the dose and frequency in the British National Formulary (BNF) book."

" Doctors carry bleeps. The bleep is a pager that wards and other doctors can ring by way of the phone system and the doctors will then ring back on the number that appears on the bleep."

" Phlebotomists go around the wards taking blood each morning. Doctors put out blood forms for them to collect the following day. Any bloods that the phlebs do not take are left for the doctor to do."

Practical Tips

Below are a few top tips from students who have been on work experience:

Introduce Yourself Do this at the start of the placement and ingratiate yourself with the team.

Patient List Ask to be given a list of patients so that you can follow who you are seeing on the ward round. Patient lists often include a brief history of the patient and will help you understand what is going on. Make sure that you give the list to one of the doctors at the end of the day or put it in the shredding bin for safe disposal, ensuring that no confidential information is allowed to leave hospital.

Gel Your Hands Squirt your hands with alcohol gel when entering or leaving a ward and if you touched a patient. Alcohol gel is effective at destroying bugs including clostridium difficile.

Watch the Foundation Doctor On ward rounds stand close to and observe the foundation doctor writing in the notes and looking at the observation charts. Be proactive and pull the curtain around the patient's bed to ensure privacy on the ward round.

Don't Worry Don't be offended if a nurse or doctor asks you to move or to do something they are simply doing their job.

Reflection: What to take from Work Experiences

From hospital work experience you need to understand what a doctor does on a daily basis and the challenges they face. Moreover by the end of your work experience you should know how they structure their day, what is good and bad about the job, what the team structure and support is like for doctors, what they do if they are unsure of anything and how they interact with other healthcare professionals.

It is also worth writing down specific things you saw such as a patient on dialysis, a man following a knee replacement, an angry relative or a patient at the end of their life. You can write down how you felt and read around the scenario, looking up how dialysis works or why a knee replacement is done.

If you witness any difficult decisions or ethical dilemmas such as a Jehovah's Witness refusing blood, a confused patient being sedated or a GP discussing contraception with a fifteen year old be sure to write these down and discuss them to understand the principles behind these tough decisions.

Chapter 4: Becoming A Doctor

Now that you are thinking about choosing medicine make sure that you know what it takes to get into medical school. This chapter gives you an idea of what is involved together with some insider tips to help you prepare.

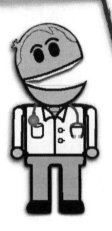

Getting Started

Entry to study medicine at university is highly competitive and, having decided to pursue a career as a doctor, the next step is to maximise your chances of selection.

Applications for medicine open through UCAS in the second week of September each year. This can be a daunting time and it is vital that you understand what is required to be successful at both application and interview and then begin preparing early to build up your knowledge and skill set to ensure success.

How to Prepare

Medical school admission boards are not just looking for academic prowess and, while it is important to gain the necessary A-Level grades, it is equally important that you present yourself as a well-rounded individual with insight into life as a doctor and a strong commitment to studying medicine.

To show that you will make a good doctor in the future you will need to demonstrate a range of extracurricular activities, work experience, voluntary experience and knowledge of medicine while achieving the required exam results at GCSE, A-Levels and on medical admission tests.

You will then need to bring all of these together in a well-written, focussed personal statement before utilising empathy, communication and reasoning skills at the medical school interview.

Doing all of this while revising for exams can seem impossible but getting started early and breaking up the steps into manageable chunks will take off much of the pressure and allow you to build yourself up and maximise your chances of selection.

Decide Chapter 1 of this book and the subsequent chapters should have given you an accurate overview of what life is like as a doctor and help you to decide.

Prepare After deciding on medicine preparing can be the most challenging step. Many students find it difficult to organise work experience and are unsure what to take from their exposure to medicine. Chapter 3 Work Experience focusses on how to gain the best experiences of medicine possible and offers tips on organising clinical and voluntary placements.

Choose Selecting a medical school is very much an individual choice and is affected by a variety of factors. Chapter 4 Choosing a Medical School and Chapter 5 The Medical School Guide guide you in your decision, offering insider tips and detailed descriptions of all UK medical schools to ensure that you have all the information required before reaching a decision.

Application Being successful at both medical school admissions tests and writing the UCAS personal statement relies on practice and insider tips. Both of these are provided in Chapter 6 Admission Tests and Chapter 7 Applying to Medical School. Graduate entry is covered in detail in Chapter 2 Graduate Entry Medicine and information on non-traditional routes such as foundation or access courses can be found later in this chapter.

Interview The key component of successful entry to medical school is the interview. Lack of preparation and insight into what interviewers look for are the main reasons individuals fall short of being offered a place. It is vital that you prepare common questions and practise giving concise answers under pressure.

Offer Hopefully you will be successful at your first time of application however if you are not you may want to consider taking a medical gap year to make your application stronger should you choose to reapply.

Timeline

Year 11

- Successfully attain GCSE grades
- Visit www.getmeintomedicalschool.com
- Look at University admissions websites
- Choose A-Levels
- Organise work experience in summer holidays
- Organise ongoing voluntary work

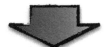

Year 12

- Successfully attain AS-Levels
- Attend University open days and choose your medical schools
- Look again at the university admissions website to see what grades they require and the format of their interview process
- Continue voluntary work
- Attend a medicine prelim course
- Successfully complete UKCAT or BMAT

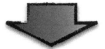

Year 13

- Submit UCAS application before October deadline
- Attend an interview practice course
- Successfully complete interviews
- Accept/decline offers

A-LEVELS

Selecting A-Level subjects appropriate for medicine and then achieving the required grades can be challenging. There are lots of factors to consider when selecting A-Levels and many myths surround the best combination of subjects and how many to take. This section aims to assist you in choosing the A-Levels that are right for you and to give you some top tips from students who have recently gained top marks in their chosen subjects.

Choosing Subjects

Choosing your A-Levels is closely linked to knowing the university course for which you wish to apply. If you are 100% certain that medicine is the career for you it is important that you are aware of the high academic requirement. The majority of medical schools ask for AAA or AAA* in science-based subjects with almost all requiring Chemistry and some requiring Biology as well. It is worth checking the admissions website of the medical schools you are considering ahead of time as entry requirements can vary dramatically between institutions. It is also advisable to consider which subjects you are good at and which you enjoy to ensure you get the best grades possible.

If you take Chemistry and Biology this will ensure that you meet the requirements of all medical schools and these subjects are often highly regarded by other courses including Law, Economics and pure science degrees if you decide to pursue something other than medicine. Topics from these two subjects appear in the early part of the medical school curriculum and mean that you will be familiar with many of the early taught concepts. We advise taking both of these subjects to A2-Level unless you have a good reason not to.

The remaining A-Levels that you choose are very much a personal choice. Physics is a popular science-based subject and topics such as gas equations, resistance and pressure are also part of the medical course and especially important in anaesthetics. Maths A-Levels are highly regarded

78

and are a viable alternative to physics. Latin is also highly regarded and, while not as useful as science subjects, will help you master anatomical terms and disease names. Languages also show diversity and will prove useful outside of medicine.

General studies and critical thinking make good 'extra' A-Levels but are not particularly well-regarded by universities and should not replace one of the above core subjects. Many medical schools do not recognise these as 'true' A-Levels and will not count them towards your application. Combinations focussing on one area such as Biology, Human Biology and Sports Science or Maths, Further Maths and Statistics can also make you seem one-dimensional and it is important that your A-Levels are balanced.

Overall we advise taking subjects that you enjoy, will get 'A' grades in and that follow the science-based guidelines.

Our top picks are:

Chemistry, Biology, Physics (+/- any other)
Chemistry, Biology, Maths (+/- any other)

How Many?

Taking three or four or more A-Levels to A-2 is very much a personal choice. Generally speaking, the more top grades you have the better, however, you do not want to take on too many subjects and most universities are happy with the basic three. Remember AAB looks much better on your UCAS form than AABD.

It is also important to be aware that some medical schools have their own scoring systems for applications which give points for the number of A grades at A-Level in science subjects and in these rare cases more may be better. Our advice is to ensure that you read up on the entry requirements and application scoring system for the universities to which you are thinking of applying.

The Medical School Guide Chapter of this book also provides information on entry and A-Level requirements for each UK medical school.

What if I Don't Take Science-Based Subjects

Some students will decide they wish to study medicine after choosing their A-Levels and some may not wish to take Biology or Chemistry. For these students it is worth looking into Access and Foundation Medical courses offered. These typically add an extra year before the start of the medical course to teach you basic sciences. More information on these courses can be found in the next section. If an Access or Foundation course is not an option you may wish to consider retaking A-Levels in science-based subjects.

Beating A-Levels

The AS and A2 years can be stressful but remember that work done throughout the year and revision for exams is worth it if you get straight As. It is important to note that medical school applications are affected by predicted A-level grades, calculated by your school from your AS results and offers are conditional on final A2 grades.

Plan to Win Creating a revision plan and noting deadlines for coursework is a great way to combat nerves and maximise your chances of doing well during the year. Visit the website of your respective exam boards such as AQA, and look at the syllabus for your chosen subjects. This will ensure that you are covering all the topics that might be tested. Give yourself plenty of time to research and edit coursework and to sit down and revise from notes and textbooks. Look through your textbooks ahead of time and divide chapters and topics up and tackle each during a set day or week of your revision timetable.

Coursework Most A-Levels are module-based with coursework forming part of your overall mark and combined with examination results. Ensuring that coursework is started early and taken seriously in class when performing experiments or writing reports in 'closed' sessions is vital. Generally speaking, your coursework should be divided into a planning and research stage where you get to grips with what is required and what examiners are looking for, the initial write-up and outline, the experiment or task and the final write-up of the conclusion and discussion. When completing your write-up ask friends and family to proof-read your draft to minimise errors and it is always useful to get the opinions of former students who may have produced similar work the previous year.

Revision Making notes throughout the year and ensuring you understand topics as they are taught is the best way to stay on top of revision. During your formal revision time look over your existing notes and both read and test yourself on important topics to ensure deep learning. Make sure you have factored in sufficient time for each subject and have covered all areas of the syllabus from both your notes and main revision text.

Past Papers Getting hold of previous years' questions is a great way to test your existing knowledge and understand the standard of knowledge the examiners are looking for. Practising questions online or from past papers will also reveal questions that are tested year after year and allow you to prepare for these in advance.

Buddy-Up Working with another student can offer a different perspective on a topic you may be finding difficult or they may have past papers that you have not yet discovered. It may also motivate you to work hard to keep up or stay ahead of your peer. The downside is that some people prefer to study alone and can be distracted from focussed revision.

It's Not All Work Make sure that you take breaks and continue to pursue your normal extracurricular activities such as sports, music and going out with friends. A set revision timetable will help to structure your time and ensure that you have time set aside to relax.

The Night Before The night before an exam can stressful and it is important that you stop revising the day before the exam and be confident in your revision. Relax, enjoy some food and get to sleep early ensuring that you have pens, pencils and equipment ready and your alarm is set for the following day.

The Exam On the day it is important to remember that being nervous is natural and you should take confidence from the fact that you have prepared properly. Read the exam instructions carefully, noting the length and how many questions need to be answered. Remember to write carefully and turn over the back page at the end. After completing the paper try not to fall into the habit of second-guessing yourself and changing your answers unless you spot an obvious mistake.

A-Level FAQs

Do Medical Schools accept A-Level Resits? This varies widely between medical schools with some happy to do so and others taking a more strict view. Try to get the best grades possible and if in doubt consult the admissions website of the medical school.

Should I get a tutor? If you are struggling in a particular subject ask yourself why? It may be that simply investing in a different textbook or asking teachers for help greatly improves your confidence. Failing this paying a tutor is a viable option. It is important to choose someone with proven success and to remember that it will still be down to your own hard work and commitment to revision and coursework.

Can I defer my entry? Again this can vary widely between medical schools and is looked at in greater detail in the gap year section. Many medical schools will not offer deferred entry owing to the competition for places but it is worth checking the admissions website or emailing the admissions department if it is not made clear.

SHOULD I TAKE A GAP YEAR?

After studying for GCSEs and A-Levels and with another five years of coursework, examinations and hard work ahead of you at medical school taking a gap year can seem extremely appealing. Taking a year out of studying is a big decision and needs to be thought about carefully. While it is a fantastic opportunity to gain exciting life experiences over a 12-month period it is also a big financial commitment and students often worry that medical schools will look on gap years unfavourably.

This chapter helps you consider the pros and cons of taking a gap year, dispels some myths about applying to medicine following a gap year and offers some ideas on where to go and what to do in your gap year.

While this section is primarily aimed at students wishing to take a Gap Year it will also be of interest to those who proceed directly to medical school and wish to travel during the long summer vacation periods.

Positives of Taking a Gap Year

There are a number a great reasons to take a gap year and many students will have strong individual feelings about taking a year out to go traveling or gain money to help pay for medical school.

Develops Maturity Going travelling, whether with others or by yourself, is a great opportunity to break free and learn to handle grown-up concepts such as budgeting, responsibility and organising trips. This will put you in good stead for the responsibility for looking after patients and dealing with challenging situations at medical school and beyond.

Life Experiences Once you enter medical school your career is on a set rail-track and a gap year may be the only time to devote a whole year to pursuing a life-goal over a prolonged timeframe. It is also a great chance to discover other cultures and open your mind to new possibilities.

Saving Money As a medical student it can be difficult to balance a part-time job with academic commitments. Working and saving money for a year can help to offset the expense of medical school.

Developing Skills Going abroad can be a fantastic opportunity to learn practical skills such as another language. Transferrable skills such as organisation, leadership and teamwork can also be developed and utilised at medical school interviews and beyond.

Doing Something Amazing From helping a charity abroad to training for a sporting event or just collecting fantastic backpacking stories will certainly impress at interviews or in the pub following lectures.

Improving Your Application It may be that you had not planned to take a gap year but were not offered a university place. A gap year can be used to boost your CV by gaining further work experience, more transferrable skills and opportunities to explore other career options to ensure that medicine is for you.

Negatives of Taking a Gap Year

While travelling is extremely exciting it can be difficult to do so on a tight budget and some individuals will be keen to continue on to university utilising their holidays and elective period to see the world.

Money While you can work during your gap year, unless you are a successful entrepreneur, it is unlikely you will be making significant money. Moreover the cost of travelling and lack of income can mean that many students rely on their families.

Being Out of Education By taking an entire 12-months out of studying it can be difficult to adjust to lectures and revising for exams.

Getting Bored Unless you have organised something worthwhile for the whole year it may be that you tire of traveling or working. You may also see your friends enjoying university life in the UK.

Going Abroad Later Most medical schools still offer plenty of time off for traveling during the summer holidays and there is also an elective period devoted to undertaking a medical placement abroad during fourth or fifth year of the medical course.

What Effect Does A Gap Year Have on My Application?

If used wisely an extra year can help to develop transferrable skills and medical work experience that will greatly improve both your personal statement and interview answers. Most universities thus look favourably on a gap year if evidence of further dedication to medicine or development of skills can be shown.

Defer or Apply after the Gap Year? There are two routes to applying to medical school with regard to taking a gap year. Either you can apply as normal during your final year of school and tick a box on the UCAS form asking for a 'deferred entry' i.e. one beginning the year after your gap year. Alternatively you can apply during your gap year. Clearly the first option gives more piece-of-mind and allows you to relax knowing you have a place at medical school waiting. However, due to the highly competitive selection process some medical schools will only defer entry for exceptional reasons. It is therefore worth looking at the individual deferring options of the medical schools that you wish to apply for.

Where Should I Go?

When thinking about a travelling one of the first questions you may ask yourself is where do I want to go?

While the traditional 'Gap Yar' is seen as a time to go backpacking and see the world in the current economic climate staying in the UK to work is also a viable option before entering university.

Europe Travelling around Europe has the advantage of being safe with relatively cheap flights and lots of landmarks to visit in major cities. Living costs can be expensive with the current Euro exchange rate and communicating can be a challenge at first before learning a second language.

USA The US is huge and there is plenty to see and do. English is the spoken language and cost of living is reasonable if on a budget with plenty of hostels and options for travellers on a budget.

Australia & New Zealand Oz is a backpacking Mecca with plenty of students travelling on trips and staying in youth hostels in Perth, Sydney, Melbourne or the Northern Territories. Similar to the US Australia is huge with plenty to do and see. New Zealand is close by and offers further natural beauty and opportunities to go bungee jumping skydiving or try other extreme sports.

Central & South America The Amazon Rain forests and Inca trail are major backpacking destinations. Crime tends to be high with tourists targeted in some poorer areas.

Africa Visiting Africa can be a very different experience depending on what you do. Most westerners fly in and out for safaris or to climb Mount Kilimanjaro and never see the poorer areas. Tanzania and Zanzibar are popular destinations and are fairly safe for students provided you stick to your travel guide. Other areas of Africa offer opportunities for charity work or to help with international projects.

South Africa Cape Town and its surroundings are very tourist friendly and offer natural beauty together with opportunities to experience extreme adventures such as shark-cage diving, skydiving and bungee jumping. Johannesburg and less well-known areas are often high in crime and less safe than the Western Cape.

China Beijing and Shanghai offer access to the north and south areas of China respectively. Incredible man-made structures such as the great wall and the terra cotta warriors offer exciting day trips and traditional architecture and temples are stunning.

Japan Often neglected due to the language barrier Japan is incredibly exciting with modern cities like Tokyo a stone's throw away from traditional Japanese temples and castles. Japan also offers ski resorts, excellent scuba diving and plenty of natural beauty together with its unique culture often exported to western society in video games and anime. Though a major business power learning Japanese is often overlooked by westerners but can prove extremely useful and stand out on your CV.

Indonesia Thailand and its surroundings are another backpacker haven with cheap accommodation and living costs combined with stunning scenery, beaches and hot climates.

Staying in the UK If you decide on taking a gap year the authors of this book encourage you to go travelling and gain life-experiences outside of the UK for a least part of your twelve months out of education. While in the UK we advise organising paid medical work experience such as working as a health care assistant (HCA), phlebotomist or summarising notes at a GP surgery. This would add to your interview ammunition and will also help pay for flights abroad. Information on these jobs can be found in the Work Experience Chapter.

What Should I Do?

Together with where to go, thinking about what to do once you get to a destination is key to making the most of your gap year.

Backpacking Clearly travelling is the major appeal to a gap year and organising a trip and seeing the world can both open your mind and develop maturity. Backpacking minimises costs and is consequently extremely popular, with tens of thousands of 18-25 year olds backpacking around the world. Due to this popularity and the rise of registered backpacking hostels, backpacking is relatively safe in most destinations. Backpacking will allow you to meet lots of like-minded individuals in hostels during your travels, share stories, stay in contact and gain perspective on life.

Developing Skills Together with developing transferrable skills a gap year also offers you the chance to learn new skills such as gaining a PADI or SSI diving certification, playing sport to a high level, learning a new language, learning to cook, learning to ski or become a ski instructor, teaching soccer or anything else that you want to try. A gap year affords you time to excel in your chosen hobby and means that it can be utilised and dipped into during future vacation periods at medical school. Skills such as languages and cooking will greatly improve your time at medical school when communicating with patients or entertaining friends.

Gain Medical Work Experience Before becoming a medical student it can be difficult enough organising medical work experience in the UK let alone in a hospital abroad. Fortunately there are some companies, such as Gap Medics (www.gapmedics.co.uk), who can organise a safe and exciting hospital placement for you outside of the UK. These placements can be expensive but will certainly give you something exciting to talk about at interview and give you an early insight into medicine in areas such as Africa, Europe or Asia.

It is equally important to continue building on your existing work experience while in the UK with further hospital placements.

Work and Make Money It is unlikely that you will be making a significant amount of money during your gap year, however, working abroad or in the UK can help to develop transferrable skills such as teamwork, communication, judgement under pressure and problem solving all of which will be useful at interview and as a doctor. By organising your gap year through a company there are often opportunities to be paid for working abroad such as teaching English abroad or running a chalet during a ski season. You can often find temporary jobs during your travels especially in Westernised countries where bar and restaurant jobs are common.

Volunteering and Charity Work International charities and projects are always looking for eager volunteers to help make a difference. Most charities will set you a target for fundraising and expect you to meet this by a set deadline. International projects such as building schools or delivering books to poorer nations rely on self-funding and though rewarding can often be a major financial burden. It is important that you do your research and are aware of the pros and cons of helping with such projects before devoting your time and money.

Things to Consider:

• Climb mountains such as Kilimanjaro	• Ski Season
	• Teach Soccer in Camp America
• Learn French, Italian, German, Spanish, Russian or Mandarin while traveling	• Bar Work in Long-Island New York
	• Life Guard in California
• Learn martial arts in China and Thailand	• Teach English in a Buddhist Monastery in Tibet
• Teach yourself computer programming and make a website or app	• Teach English and Cricket in South Africa
• Trek to the North Pole	• Work as a groundsman and teach rugby in Canada
• Complete the Inca Trail	
• Cycle to Rome for charity	• Backpack around Europe, Thailand, Australia
• Do an Army/Navy/RAF paid gap year before going to Sandhurst after med school	• Road trip across USA

Plan Your Trip Research, research and research is key to making the most of your gap year. Search the web and buy books on gap year travel together with talking with friends and family who may have done similar trips.

Think about whether you want to do part or all of your trip solo or with friends and include them in the planning stage.

Budget When planning your trip write down how much you can afford to spend and then write out the cost of flights, accommodation, Visas and daily food and drink budget to give you an idea of how much you need to save.

Organise Visas Some countries offer reciprocal access to the UK such as Europe, USA or Japan others require that you apply for a tourist or working visa. It is important that you check visa requirements with the corresponding embassy website well in advance as some visa applications can take upwards of four weeks to process.

Book Flights Early By organising flights outside of popular times and flying midweek you may be able to make significant savings on flights. Some websites such as STA Travel also offer discounts for students and offer ideas for trips and connections.

Get Immunisations and Vaccinations If you are going to tropical areas such as Africa, South America or Indonesia it is important to check their embassy websites to see if the country requires immunisations against endemic diseases such as yellow fever. If you are undertaking medical work experience abroad you will also need to have records of up-to-date Hep-B, C and TB vaccinations. Most hospitals or companies will be able to guide you on what is required.

Medical Application If you have not succeeded in deferring your entry ensure that you will be back in the UK for medical school interview dates and that all your medical-related experiences happen before the interview date to maximise what you can talk about to interviewers.

FOUNDATION AND ACCESS COURSES

If you have decided to study medicine after selecting non-science A-Levels there are still a number of options available for applying to medical school.

Foundation or Premed Courses

Foundation or 'Premed' courses are designed to give students without science A-Levels a year of science teaching before commencing the standard undergraduate course. They are effectively a six-year medical course with guaranteed progression onto the medical course after completion of the Foundation year.

There are 13 UK Medical Schools that offer Foundation courses. Competition for places is fierce and you still need to attain AAA in your non-science A-Levels to receive an offer.

Students apply for the premed/foundation course through UCAS and following one year of full time study at the university students are guaranteed a place on the undergraduate medical course.

Premed/Foundation Courses:

• Bristol	• Nottingham
• Durham	• Norwich: UEA
• Keele	• Sheffield
• Leeds (At Bradford)	• Southampton
• Liverpool	• Cardiff
• London: King's	• Dundee
• Manchester	

Access Courses

Some institutions that do not have a medical school run medical access courses. These are primarily designed for mature students to demonstrate recent academic activity, though some can help to augment those who received poor A-level grades.

Many medical schools do not recognise access courses and, unlike foundation courses, there is no guaranteed place at a medical school following their completion. Make sure you check with both the access course and your prospective medical school that the course is recognised before you apply.

Access Courses:

- City & Islington College, London

- City College Norwich, Norfolk

- College of West Anglia, Norfolk (Linked with UEA Medical School)

- Lambeth College, London

- The Manchester College, Manchester

- St Martin's College, Lancashire

- Sussex Downs College, East Sussex (Linked with Brighton & Sussex Medical School)

FINANCES

Medicine is a five year course and it is important that you are aware of the magnitude of debt that you will be taking onboard together with the options available for funding and how this debt affects you following graduation.

It is not all doom and gloom however as in the final year of your medical course you will be entitled to a non-repayable NHS bursary covering tuition fees and a means-tested maintenance. Student loans cover most costs and are repayable at a low rate of interest following graduation.

Tuition fees and maintenance student loans vary depending on where you come from in the UK.

To help you understand the facts and figures this section divides student loans into England, Scotland, Wales, Northern Ireland and International based on where you live.

We then look at other sources of financial support and budgeting as a student before taking you through how your loan will be repaid.

Tuition fees

For UK and EU students the maximum fee charged by a UK university is £9,000 in 2015. The exact amount may vary between different universities but all universities clearly show course fees on their websites. International students are often charge different fees for studying in the UK and if you have studied a prior university course, this may affect the level of support you are entitled to.

It is advisable to apply for student finance when the cycle begins in spring to guarantee that funds are deposited in your account for the course start date.

Tuition Fee Loans

I am from England

You will need to apply to Student Finance England for a loan to cover your tuition fees. This loan is not means tested and The Student Loans Company (SLC) pays your tuition fees directly to your university.

To ensure that the loan amount is in place for the start date of your course note that the deadline for applications to Student Finance England is the end of April each year.

After you have graduated you will start repaying your loan once you are earning more than £21,000 per year.

I am from Wales

You will apply to Student Finance Wales for a loan of up to £3,575. A Fee Grant will pay the balance of the tuition fee up to a maximum grant of £5,425 if a tuition fee of £9,000 is charged.

The deadline for applications to Student Finance Wales to guarantee that funds are in place for the beginning of the academic year is the beginning of April each year.

After you have graduated you will start repaying your loan once you are earning more than £21,000 per year.

I am from Scotland

You will apply to the Student Awards Agency for Scotland (SAAS) for a loan to cover your tuition fees.

The deadline date for applications to SAAS to guarantee that funds are in place for the beginning of the academic year is the end of March each year.

After you have graduated you will start repaying your loan once you are earning over £16,365 a year.

I am from Northern Ireland

You will apply to Student Finance NI for a loan to cover your tuition fees.

The deadline date for applications to Student Finance NI to guarantee that funds are in place for the beginning of the academic year is the beginning of April each year.

After you have graduated you will start repaying your loan once you are earning over £16,365 a year.

I am an international student

International students normally resident in countries outside the EU and EEA pay near-full-cost tuition fees in all the UK universities.

Maintenance (Living Costs) Loans

I am from England

Maintenance Loan You will need to apply to Student Finance England for a means-tested maintenance loan. The maximum maintenance loan for students is £7,675 if you live away from home and study in London, £5,500 if you live away from home and study outside London and £4,375 if you choose to live at home.

Maintenance Grant You may also apply for a grant if your family income is below £42,611. You are eligible for a maintenance grant of £3,354 if your household income is < £25,000 and slightly less if your household income is between £25,000 and £42,611.

Other Options Further support may be available to certain categories of students such as lone parents, those with dependants and those leaving care to enter higher education. Extra help is also available to those who have a disability, learning difficulty or mental health problem.

I am from Wales

Maintenance Loan You will need to apply to Student Finance Wales for a means-tested maintenance loan. The maximum available is £7,215 if you are living and studying in London, £5,150 if you are living and studying outside London and £3,987 if you are living at home. You may also be able to receive a partial cancellation of up to £1,500 on your living cost (maintenance) loan, subject to the approval of the National Assembly for Wales.

Assembly Learning Grant (ALG) You may be eligible for the full grant of £5,161 a year if your household income is £18,370 a year or less. A partial grant of between £50 and £5,000 a year is payable if your household income is between £18,371 and £50,020.

Other Options Further support may be available to certain categories of students such as lone parents, those with dependants and those leaving care to enter higher education. Extra help is also available to those who have a disability, learning difficulty or mental health problem.

I am from Scotland

SAAS Loan You will need to apply to the Student Awards Agency Scotland (SAAS) for a means-tested loan of up to £5,500.

Young Student's Bursary This reduces the SAAS loan by a maximum of £1,750 a year if your family income is £16,999 or less a year.

Other Options Supplementary grants are available to certain categories of students such as lone parents, those with dependants and those leaving care to enter higher education. Extra help is also available to those who have a disability, learning difficulty or mental health problem.

I am from Northern Ireland

Maintenance Loan You will need to apply to Student Finance NI for a means-tested maintenance loan. The maximum available is £6,780 if you are living and studying in London, £4,840 if you are living and studying outside London and £3,750 if you are living at home.

Maintenance Grant If your household income is £41,065 or less you may be eligible to receive a maintenance grant. A full grant is worth £3,475 and is payable if your total household income is £19,203 or less.

Other Options Supplementary grants are available to certain categories of students such as lone parents, those with dependents and those leaving care to enter higher education. Extra help is also available to those who have a disability, learning difficulty or mental health problem.

Other Sources of Funding

University Bursaries and Scholarships

Many universities offer scholarships or bursaries to students who meet set criteria. This might be a sports scholarship, an academic scholarship or a hardship bursary. The number, type and amount offered varies widely between universities and it is worth looking at the finance website of your chosen universities to see if you qualify for a bursary or scholarship.

NHS Bursary

Standard 5-Year Course From year five onwards your tuition fees will be paid by the NHS Student Bursary Scheme and you will be eligible to apply for a means-tested NHS bursary to cover maintenance costs and a reduced maintenance loan from Student Finance England.

GEM Programmes Graduates on accelerated courses are eligible for a lower NHS bursary from the second year of the course. The NHS Bursary scheme will pay £3,465 towards your tuition fees from year two with student loan covering the remaining amount.

Professional and Career-Development Loans

If you are really struggling some high-street banks offer loans up to £10, 000 which are repayable upon graduation. The interest on these loans tends to be higher than the student loan and may greatly eat into your pay cheques.

Armed Forces Cadetships

If you are interested in a career as a medic in the armed forces there are a number of funding options. The drawback is that you will be required to undertake foundation jobs in army hospitals (usually around Birmingham) and will be enlisted to serve for around 6 years.

Army Medic The Undergraduate Cadetship offers a chance for future doctors, who pass officer selection, to earn money while studying for a degree. The Army will pay your tuition fees and you will also get an annual salary of around £14,515 for the last three years of your course.

Medical students will also have the chance to do work on attachment at Army medical units, either in the UK or overseas. In return you'll be expected to serve for six years after you've qualified and completed officer training.

To be eligible you must be a British, Commonwealth or Irish citizen studying at a UK university, within three years of finishing your course.

Royal Air Force Medic Medical Bursars receive a maximum bursary of £6,000 payable in years 2 and 3 then compete for the Cadetship upgrade for years 4 and 5.

You'll also get the chance to join the University Air Squadron (UAS), where you'll get an excellent experience of how life in the RAF works, including learning to fly, going on ski expeditions and being involved in aeromedical evacuations.

Royal Navy Medic The sponsorship package includes a salary of £14,301 rising to £17,881, tuition fees, London allowance (if applicable), book allowance of £50 per annum, overseas medical electives and opportunity to take advantage of all sport and adventure training facilities.

During your degree you will have the opportunity to be a member of one of the University Royal Navy Units. After graduating you will complete the two year foundation programme in one of the Ministry Defence Hospital Units (MDHUs) in Portsmouth, Plymouth, Frimley Park, Peterborough or Birmingham.

Saving Money During Medical School

Budgeting and ensuring that you keep on top of your finances is our most important tip. Ensure that you know when your student loan enters you account and when bills for rent, mobile phone and gym membership are withdrawn. Mobile banking apps and online banking make your account instantly accessible.

Students are also eligible for a wealth of offers from high street chains, online stores and travel companies and it is important to be aware that just by being a student you may qualify for a discount. The 16-25 railcard reduces your rail fares by one third and is a great way to take your washing home after a long semester.

Working Your Way Through Medical School

Getting a part-time job is a great source of income to help fund your degree course or pay for summer holidays. Jobs can also help to improve transferrable skills such as teamwork, communication and leadership. Other jobs such as bar work can be sociable and allow you to meet people outside of the medical course. You could even work as a phlebotomist or healthcare assistant at a local hospital to help gain further insight into life on the wards.

Top Uni Jobs

Club Event Promoter Bars and clubs will often pay handsomely if you can persuade students to attend their student nights. This can be hard work but if you create a weekly club night it is likely that you will make yourself a tidy profit.

Bar Work Working in bars and pubs can be busy but also offers the opportunity to meet new people and socialise.

HCA/Phlebotomist Paying between £6.50-£10/hour these are good options that will also look good on your CV. The downside is that shifts can be long and washing and feeding patients or taking blood may not be for everyone.

Cold-Caller for University Most universities pay students to cold-call graduates to see if they would like to donate to the university. This typically pays around £8 per hour and provided you don't mind being hung-up on is fairly easy money.

Entrepreneur If you are business-minded or IT literate there is nothing stopping you from creating the new Angry Birds or selling a product over the internet. Many savvy students spot opportunities to help their fellow students while making some money too.

Once You Graduate

Your first pay packet will not be taxed and this will equate to taking home around £2200 in your first month of work. As an F1 you will likely be taking home between £1600-2000 per month depending on your job banding and the hospital that you work in.

National insurance, Tax and NHS pension will be automatically deducted from your payslip. National insurance is around £300 per month, Tax is around £500 per month and NHS pension is around £200 per month for an FY1 doctor.

In England and Wales once you are earning greater than £21,000 your student loan will also be deducted from your payslip as 9% of your income. In Scotland and Northern Ireland this figure is £16,365. This equates to around £200 per month automatically deducted from your monthly pay packet.

This will leave you with between £1000-1500 to spend on rent and whatever else you wish to buy.

Your salary jumps up following completion of F1 with F2 doctors taking home £2000-2400. There are also opportunities to do extra shifts as a locum doctor once you reach F2. Typical locum rates are £25-35 per hour.

Useful links

- Student Finance England
- Student Finance Wales
- Student Awards Agency for Scotland (SAAS)
- Student Finance NI

Chapter 5: Graduate Entry Medicine (GEM)

Graduate entry and mature medics have the advantage of knowing the amount of work required to do well at university and, having already experienced the highs of Freshers' week and first year, may be keen to get down to business from the outset.

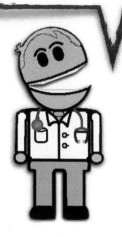

MAKING THE DECISION

Choosing to undertake a four or five year degree course after completing a previous degree can be a difficult decision. Not only do gradate and mature students face another lengthy period of study they must also deal with the financial and social implications of returning to University.

Graduate and Mature Entry Options

Graduate Entry Medicine (GEM) A few medical schools offer an accelerated 4-year medical degree for graduates. These tend to be popular as the NHS bursary extends to cover three years of the GEM course rather than just the last year on the standard 5-year course. To shorten the course topics from the first two years are combined leading to a heavier workload and a more stressful exam period for GEM students. For the remaining years, graduate entry courses and undergraduate courses are often the same. (More information can be found in the GEM section).

Mature Entry Medicine GEM programmes are not the only way for mature students to get into medical school. You may also apply for standard five (or six) year undergraduate courses. Many medical schools have a small number of places reserved for mature students, although some do not allow graduates onto their undergraduate course, preferring them to apply to their GEM course only (Nottingham and St. George's are examples).

Things to Consider

Together with the entry options mature and graduate students face all the same decisions as undergraduates plus a few more.

Age Medical schools do not have an upper age limit, and there are plenty of students in their thirties studying medicine. It is important to remember that the course is at least four years in length and if you apply to GP (which has the shortest postgraduate training) it will still be five years until you become a partner following graduation. Think about whether you will be able to cope with on calls, night shifts and taking instructions from seniors younger than you.

Family and Dependents Returning to full-time study, particularly if you are employed, can greatly affect your family. Make sure you talk through the decision with your partner and/or children and that they understand that you will be rotating around hospitals, working shifts and taking on extra debt. You may have to relocate for medical school and then again for postgraduate posts depending on how you fare at job applications.

Cost Tuition fees currently stand at £9,000 per year and this will add to any existing debts you may have. Graduates on GEM courses are offered a three year NHS Bursary compared to graduates on a standard course who are offered only one year. Further info on GEM finances can be found in the GEM Courses section.

Entry Requirements

Most medical schools place more weight on your most recent degree than on your GCSE or A-Level grades and a 2:1 is considered the minimum standard for both standard and GEM courses.

The types of degrees that medical schools accept varies widely with some only accepting graduates from science backgrounds while others are opening their doors to graduates with any degree.

Work experience is even more important for graduates. Some medical schools want graduates from non-health care backgrounds to have at least four months experience working as a healthcare assistant or similar.

A-Levels These are less important than for undergraduates but some medical schools still require Chemistry or Biology. Make sure you carefully check the requirements of your chosen medical schools and decide whether you want to sit an extra A-Level or apply somewhere with different required subjects.

Access Courses If you are a mature student and have been out of education for more than three years access courses can help to demonstrate an ongoing commitment to studying. They are not accepted by all medical schools and it is important to check the respective admission website or email the admissions department directly before signing up to a yearlong access course.

Admission Tests Graduates applying to both the standard and GEM courses may be required to sit the UKCAT, BMAT or GAMSAT. Don't assume that the admission test requirements will be the same as for school leavers and make sure you read the graduate-specific test requirements for both the standard and GEM courses.

GEM COURSES

Graduate Entry Medicine (GEM) courses are accelerated four-year medical courses for students with a previous degree. The courses assume a level of maturity and the ability to adapt quickly to the work load. GEM courses are appealing as they allow for completion of the medical degree in a shorter time and with less debt.

Graduates can also apply to the standard five year courses and making the choice between the accelerated GEM courses and the standard medical course can be tough.

GEM Advantages

Shorter Course Length Having already completed a degree course you will be eager to graduate and start working and earning in the real world with your peers.

Money A four year course will save you £9,000 on tuition fees plus any accommodation and maintenance expenses. You will also be earning money a year sooner and receive more NHS support (see below).

Bursary Graduates on GEM courses are entitled to an NHS bursary for years 2-4 of the accelerated course. Graduates on standard courses are only entitled to an NHS bursary for their final year.

Peers The Swansea and Warwick GEM courses are graduate only and GEM courses at other universities tend to keep graduates in their own groups. This will allow you to work with fellow graduates in an environment less dominated by school leavers.

Focus on Degree The selection process to GEM courses places less weighting on GCSEs and A-Levels and more on your most recent degree. This can be an advantage if you did not do as well as you would have liked at GCSE and A-Levels.

GEM Disadvantages

Limited Medical Schools There are a limited number of medical schools offering GEM courses which may restrict where you can apply.

Competitive GEM courses tend to be popular with graduates and it can be difficult to stand out in the selection process.

Small Size GEM intakes tend to be small and you will be attending your lectures and tutorials with the same small group of peers.

Hard Work To shorten the medical course the first two GEM years are often extremely busy with a plethora of lectures and tutorials to attend and the scope of information to revise for examinations can seem overwhelming.

GEM Finances

Year One

In Year 1 you will be charged an annual tuition fee, which in 2015 is £9,000. GEM students are responsible for paying the first £3,465 of this amount to the University themselves. Eligible students can apply for a tuition fee loan from Student Finance England (SFE) for the remainder of the fee £5,535. This loan is not means tested.

You may be eligible to take out a loan towards living costs from SFE of up to £5,500. 65% of this amount is non means tested, the remaining £35% is means tested on household income.

Apply on-line for both the Tuition Fee Loan and the Loan for Living Costs at www.gov.uk/studentfinance .

You will not be entitled to receive a grant towards living costs, but depending on your circumstances you may be eligible for supplementary grants e.g. Adult Dependants Grant; Childcare Grant, from SFE.

Years Two, Three and Four

In years two to four the NHS will pay the first £3,465 (or equivalent) towards the University tuition fee. For the remaining amount you will be able to apply to Student Finance England for a tuition fee loan.

To help with living costs you may receive a non means tested Grant of £1,000, plus a means tested Bursary from the NHS. The maximum bursary for a 30 week academic year is £2,591. A further £82 per week is available for any week above the 30. A lower rate Bursary is offered if you live with your parents during term time.

In addition you may be eligible for a non means tested loan of £2,324 (£1,744 if you live with your parents) from Student Finance England.

You may be eligible for supplementary grants e.g. Dependants Allowance; Childcare Allowance, from the NHS.

Chapter 6: Admission Tests

The UKCAT, BMAT and GAMSAT are used to help universities differentiate between candidates who may all have top (predicted) A-Levels. Different universities require different tests and the key to getting a good score is to practice.

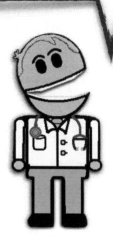

A Guide to Admission Tests

Medical school admissions tests were devised as a way to help medical admission boards distinguish between candidates with similar predicted a-levels, standardise testing and level the playing field for applicants from struggling schools.

Their use remains controversial and research published in medical education journals is divided on whether they help select the best future doctors or not.

Whether they are useful or not, the majority of UK medical schools require admissions testing as part of their application and if you wish to apply to one of these institutions admissions tests are something you will need to do.

There are three admission tests used by UK medical schools:

- **UK Clinical Aptitude Test (UKCAT)** this is widely used and consists of five sections: verbal reasoning, quantitive reasoning, abstract reasoning, decision analysis and non-cognitive analysis.

- **BioMedical Admissions Test (BMAT)** this is needed for Oxbridge, Imperial, UCL and graduate entry at Brighton Sussex. It consists of three sections: aptitude and skills, scientific knowledge and applications and the writing task.

- **Graduate Medical School Admissions Test (GAMSAT)** this is needed for graduate entry courses at Exeter, St George's, Nottingham, Peninsula and Swansea medical schools. It consists of three sections: reasoning in humanities and social science, written communication, reasoning in biological and physical science.

Birmingham, Bristol and Liverpool medical schools do not require any admissions tests and are satisfied with the traditional, tried and tested method of selecting future doctors.

You must pay to sit each of the tests and you only get one chance with no re-sits offered. The format of each admissions test differs and they are very different from A-Level examinations.

While the examiners of admissions tests claim that no revision is necessary familiarising yourself with the format and timing of the questions is a vital component of being successful. Carefully reading their websites and completing timed practise papers will help you to understand what the examiners are looking for and is the best way to prepare.

In this chapter we will help you understand how medical schools use these tests in the admissions process, outline which universities want which tests, give you an overview of the best ways to prepare and then look at each individual test in detail.

How Medical Schools Use Admissions Tests

As you will read later on in this book the medical application process is not standardised and varies significantly between each university. While some medical schools are open about how admissions test scores contribute to your application others prefer not to divulge precisely how mark ranges are scored or test results weighted. Some have a set cut off for UKCAT, BMAT or GAMSAT scores with only candidates above the cut off called for interview while others assign their own scores to mark-ranges and add these scores to candidates' overall application score.

Preparing for Admissions Tests

Once you have decided which admissions test you need to take the next step is deciding when and where you will take them.

Each test costs a slightly different amount and takes place at a different time of year as you will see below. Be sure to register early to avoid missing any deadlines. The below table highlights key dates, it is also important to check the individual websites as deadlines may change if there are difficulties with test centres or the registration system.

Admissions Test Deadlines

	UKCAT	BMAT	GAMSAT
Cost	£65-80	£44	£228
Registration Opens	1st May	1st September	3rd June
Registration Closes	20th September	1st October	9th August
Deadline for Payment	On Booking	15th October	9th August
Test Date	1st July – 4th October	6th November	18th September
Results Date	Same day as test	27th November	End of November

Understanding the Format and Practising

After registering the next step is to understand the format of the individual test.

While you will not be able to revise facts and principles in the same way you will be doing for A-Levels practicing past papers will give you a better understanding of the pacing of the test, the type of questions asked and how these questions are marked.

A recent study at a British university using current doctors as subjects found that those who had undertaken a practice admission test did significantly better than those who had not when taking the final test.

You can find information on the individual test components in the later sections of this chapter looking at each admission test in turn. Below are some suggested ways to prepare for admissions tests:

School Some schools run sessions on doing well at admissions test. Teachers are also a good resource for offering feedback on your essay writing or might be able to suggest books or local courses that can help.

This Book By reading this chapter and trying the sample questions you will get a good idea of what admissions tests require and what areas you may find difficult. Recent students also offer top tips on doing well.

Admission Test Websites All three admission tests have websites featuring the latest information on the format and timing for each test. They also offer sample questions and tips for doing well.

Question Books There are several books available featuring pure test questions to practice. These are useful for the UKCAT and BMAT knowledge questions but will be unable to offer individualised feedback on essay questions. It is important that you ensure books contain comprehensive explanations for each answer, as this is the most important way to learn.

Online Question Banks Several website offer online question banks with practice questions. These usually cost around £30 for unlimited access. Kaplan is the most well known but is expensive.

Courses and Tutoring While practising is the most important way to learn, if you are struggling attending an admissions test course or hiring a tutor is another viable option. Courses will often offer tips and explain how to answer questions, the downside is that these can be expensive and do not guarantee success.

Reading Around Some admission test books explain how to do well in each of the test specific components, however, if you are struggling in a specific component it may be worth reading around an area. A pure abstract reasoning text or a math book may give you some extra tips or an alternative perspective to tackling questions.

Improving Your Technique

Each test has different sections testing different components. While some components, such as the UKCAT's quantitive reasoning, test skills you will have developed at school such as maths, others may seem very bizarre, such as the UKCAT's abstract reasoning, and it can be difficult to identify what examiners consider to be a correct answer.

Remember that there is only one correct answer and when an answer is not obvious it is down to technique and a process of elimination to choose what the examiners consider to be the best choice.

If you have already attempted some practice questions you may have already identified areas of personal weakness. For example you may be a natural at abstract reasoning but struggle under pressure with math calculations. We recommend focusing on your areas of weakness and utilising some of the previous resources and below tips to improve your chances of success.

Practice Questions Do as many practice questions as possible, practice is key. Question books and online question banks provide plenty and will help you to understand what examiners are looking for and also to identify areas that you struggle with. We also suggest trying doing mock tests to time to help with your time management.

Understanding Timing The times for each exam are listed in their individual section below. Timing is tight and it is important you are aware of how long you have to answer questions in each section. The UKCAT gives you around 30 seconds per question which means there is very little thinking time and if you are unsure of answer it is best to make an educated guess and go with your gut rather than lose time trying to work it out.

Best-Guessing The multiple-choice question format is not negatively marked and thus you are not punished for wrong answers. You will definitely score zero on a question if you do not answer it but have a 1 in 4 or 1 in 5 chance of getting it right if you put down an answer. You will not be 100%

sure of every answer and the abstract nature of certain questions necessitates eliminating answers that are clearly wrong which often leaves you with a 50-50 chance.

Don't Dwell on Long or Tough Questions Often referred to as question triage (triage being French for sorting), by quickly answering the short more straightforward questions and guessing or skipping the longer or tougher questions you will ensure you reach the end of the section component within the time. We would recommend ensuring you are aware of timings as mentioned above and putting down a best guess for tough or long questions. You should note down the questions you triage, as you may have time to come back to them at the end.

Written Answers The BMAT features a written component and it is important that your handwriting is legible and that you structure you answers in a logical manner to facilitate marking. The examiners will have a set mark sheet and by structuring your points with paragraphs or headings you will improve your overall score.

Taking the Test

As with any exam you take handling nerves and remembering your preparation are key. Below are a few tips to help you during the testing period.

The Night Before Ensure that you get a good night's sleep. There is no knowledge or syllabus to cram in the preceding days and if you have practised questions well in advance and understand what the examiners are looking you should take confidence from your preparation. Plan what you wish to take; a watch, calculator and spare pens and pencils are a good start.

The Test Centre Access the website for the admissions test that you are taking and make sure you know what time you need to be at the test centre, how long it will take to get there and what you need to take with you. The website also give plans of how the test centres are laid out with space to store your coat and bag and a layout of the seating.

Test Day Make sure that you get up, have breakfast and leave in good time to reduce nerves. If you are very worried it may be worth doing a test run to the centre a few days before the exam so you know where you are going on the day. Report to the reception area and then take your seat. Remember to switch off your mobile phone.

The Test Remain calm and remember your timings. You should know how long you can spend on each question, if any questions are very long or tough don't let them phase you, make a guess and move on, coming back later if you have time. Basic exam mantras such as read the question, tick the correct box, write clearly and check your answers should be running through your mind. For written papers it may be useful to highlight or underline key words to help you focus on the question, for computer-based tests reading carefully is key.

After the Test Do not dwell on any questions, relax knowing that you have given it your best shot and wait for the results.

THE UKCAT

There are two versions of UKCAT: the standard UKCAT and the UKCATSEN (Special Educational Needs). The UKCATSEN is a longer version of the UKCAT intended for candidates who require additional time due to a documented medical condition or disability. The timings of the two tests are detailed below:

Section	Questions	Standard Test Time	Extended Test Time
Verbal Reasoning	44	22 minutes	28 minutes
Quantitative Reasoning	36	23 minutes	29 minutes
Abstract Reasoning	65	16 minutes	20 minutes
Decision Analysis	26	32 minutes	40 minutes
Situational Judgment Test	60*	27 minutes	33 minutes

*13 scenarios (each consisting of between 4 and 6 potential response options to rate)

Verbal Reasoning

Assesses your logical thinking and reasoning about written information. You must select whether each statement is: 'True', 'False' or 'Can't Tell' using only the information provided in the passage. The key to this section is reading the information at face value and not assuming any information.

Questions: 44 (11 passages with 4 questions per passage) lasting 22 minutes.

Timing: 2 minutes per passage, 30 seconds per question

Quantitative Reasoning

Assesses your ability to solve numerical problems and quickly extrapolate information from charts, graphs and tables.

Questions: 36 (9 sets of tables/graphs/charts with 4 questions each) lasting 23 minutes.

Timing: Approximately 2.5 minutes per table/chart/graph, 30 seconds per question

Abstract Reasoning

Assesses the use of convergent and divergent thinking to infer relationships from information. You are presented with two 'sets' of shapes labeled 'Set A' and 'Set B'. Each set has a 'rule' or common factor which links all the shapes in their corresponding set. You must assign a test shape to Set A, B or neither.

Questions: 65 (13 pairs of sets, 5 test shapes to assign to one of each pair) lasting 16 minutes

Timing: Approximately 1 minute per pair of sets

Decision Analysis

Assesses the ability, in complex, ambiguous situations, to deal with various forms of information, infer relationships, make informed judgments and decide on an appropriate response. You will be asked to decipher a code using an algorithm that can be interpreted in a number of ways. Each question will have several options and you must choose the most appropriate translated code.

Questions: 26 (separate question but overall code used is often the same)

Timing: Approximately 1 minute per question

Situational Judgment Test

Assesses judgment regarding situations encountered in the workplace. You will be asked to read a short scenario and then choose the course of action that you believe is most appropriate. This section tests empathy, integrity and professionalism together with judgment.

Questions: 60 (13 scenarios with 4-6 responses to choose from) lasting 27 minutes

Timing: Approximately 2 minutes per scenario, 20 seconds per question

UKCAT Top Tips

Below are a few top tips from candidates who were successful at the UKCAT.

Take The Test Early Getting it out of the way will allow you to concentrate on other things (such as your UCAS application!). If you book early you will have your choice of test slots and if you then feel unwell or unprepared you will have an opportunity to reschedule. This might not be easy in the final weeks of testing.

Only One Right Answer Good multiple-choice questions include answer options that are wrong but seem almost right. Work hard to find them and eliminate them. Questions like these are not tricks. Accept that one (and only one) of the answers to each question is correct

Don't Panic Many candidates do not complete all sections in the test. Use the practice test to ensure you know how to pace yourself. Try to answer all the questions but don't worry if you don't get to the end of each section.

Don't Leave Blanks There is a point for each right answer, but no points are deducted for wrong answers. Try not to leave blanks. If you really can't work out the answer, it is better to eliminate the answers that you know to be wrong and then make your best guess from those that are left. If you are struggling with a question move on to the next one. You can mark questions for review so that you can skip them and come back to them later.

THE BMAT

Cambridge, London: Imperial, London: UCL and Oxford undergraduate courses and the Brighton Sussex Graduate entry course require the Biomedical Admissions Test (BMAT).

Results for the BMAT last only for the year you apply and you can re-sit the test should you reapply.

The BMAT is a pen and paper, written test composed of three sections and lasts two hours.

Section	Questions	Timing
Aptitude and Skills	35 (MCQ and short answers)	60 minutes
Scientific Knowledge and Application	27 (MCQ and short answers)	30 minutes
Writing Task	1 essay from a choice of 4	30 minutes

Aptitude and Skills

A 60-minute section consisting of 35 multiple-choice or short answer questions. It tests generic skills often used in undergraduate study, including:

Problem Solving: 13 marks are available for your ability to select relevant information, recognise similarities and apply simple numerical and algebraic algorithms to solve problems.

Understanding Argument: 10 marks are available for your ability to reason, make assumptions and draw conclusions from a series of logical arguments.

Data Analysis and Inference Abilities: 12 marks are available for your ability to interpret and reach conclusions from information presented in text, tables and graphs.

Timing: Approximately 1.5 minutes per question

Scientific Knowledge and Application

A 30-minute section consisting of 27 multiple-choice or short answer questions. It is restricted to material normally encountered in non-specialist Science and Mathematics (i.e. up to and including National Curriculum Key Stage 4 Science and Mathematics). The section is more concerned about the application of principles rather than the core facts taught in GCSE maths and science.

Questions: The 27 MCQs are equally divided (6-8 in each) between biology, chemistry, physics and maths.

Timing: Approximately 1 minute per question

Writing Task

A 30-minute section consisting of four essay questions, of which the candidate must answer only one.

The writing task asks you to form a well-written coherent argument on the subject proposed. You are limited to a single side of A4 and it is vital that you spend 5-10 minutes planning your essay as up to 20% of marks are awarded for organisation and structure of the essay.

Questions: Essay questions are marked by two examiners. Each examiner gives two scores – one for quality of content (on a scale of 0–5), and one for quality of written English (on the scale A, C, E).

Timing: 30 minutes

BMAT Top Tips

Below are some top tips from students who have passed the BMAT.

Practise The BMAT website offers past paper questions and practice questions. As with the UKCAT understanding the timings and how the questions are presented is key to doing well.

Plan the Essay Think about how you will divide up and structure your essay. Use scrap paper to jot down bullet points and ideas that you can incorporate into your final work.

Use Personal Examples Using personal examples is a great way to make your essay interesting for the marker and also shows that you can relate the assignment to the wider world.

Write Clearly As a future doctor it is assumed that your handwriting is illegible. Try to make sure your essay is neatly written and that the marker can easily read it.

Check Your Spelling Grammatical and spelling errors can make you look foolish, make sure you factor in time at the end of the essay section to read over your work.

THE GAMSAT

The GAMSAT is used for graduate-entry courses at Keele, London: St. George's, Nottingham and Swansea.

A full day is needed to sit the GAMSAT. The test is made up of five and a half (5½) hours of testing time and one hour of break time. Ten minutes reading time is given for Sections I and III and five minutes for Section II.

Section	Questions	Timing
Reasoning in Humanities and Social Sciences	75	100 minutes
Written Communication	2	60 minutes
Reasoning in Biological and Physical Sciences	110	170 minutes

Reasoning in Humanities and Social Sciences

This section tests skills in the interpretation and understanding of ideas in social and cultural contexts. Different kinds of text are used, including passages of personal, imaginative, expository and argumentative writing. Although most of the materials in this section are in the form of written passages, some units may present ideas and information in visual and tabular form. Materials deal with a range of academic and public issues, with an emphasis on socio-cultural, personal and interpersonal topics.

Timing: 1 minute 20 seconds per question

Written Communication

This section is a test of your ability to produce and develop ideas in writing. It involves two thirty-minute writing tasks. Each task offers a number of ideas relating to a common theme. The first task deals with socio-cultural issues while the second deals with more personal and social issues. Each piece of writing is assessed by three markers who award marks in two domains: Thought and Content (what is said) and Organisation and Expression (the structure and language used).

Timing: 30 minutes per written task

Reasoning in Biological and Physical Sciences

Material is presented in a variety of formats including text, numbers, graphs, tables and diagrams. Along with testing reasoning and problem solving within a scientific context, this section examines the recall and understanding of basic science concepts.

The level of subject knowledge required generally corresponds to the first year of university studies in biology and chemistry, and Leaving Certificate or A-level in physics.

Questions: 110 four-stemmed multiple choice questions test your knowledge of Chemistry (40%), Biology (40%) and Physics (20%).

Timing: 1 minute 30 seconds per question

GAMSAT Top Tips

Below are some top tips from graduates who have successfully passed the GAMSAT.

It's a Marathon Make sure you take food and drink and use the rest periods wisely. The exam will be tiring and it is important that you remain focussed and at your best.

Brush Up On Your Sciences If you have not come from a science degree you will need to make sure you practise the science-based questions and read up on any topics that you are unsure about.

Plan the Essay Think about how you will divide up and structure your essay. Use scrap paper to jot down bullet points and ideas that you can incorporate into your final work.

Use Personal Examples Using personal examples is a great way to make your essay interesting for the marker and also shows that you can relate the assignment to the wider world.

Write Clearly As a future doctor it is assumed that your handwriting is illegible. Try to make sure your essay is neatly written and that the marker can easily read it.

Check Spelling Grammatical and spelling errors can make you look foolish, make sure you factor in time at the end of the essay section to read over your work.

We hope you found the book useful and wish you luck in your medical school application.

Also In The Get Me Into Medical School! Series:

1. Should I Become A Doctor?

2. Choose A Medical School

3. The Medical School Interview

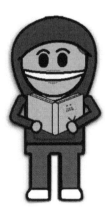

For the latest information be sure to check out

www.getmeintomedicalschool.com

And follow us on Twitter

www.twitter.com/getmeintomed

Made in the USA
San Bernardino, CA
25 November 2017